CENTERS FOR MEDICARE & MEDICAID SERVICES

Medicare & You

2012

This is the **official U.S. government** Medicare handbook:

 Open Enrollment now begins October 15 and ends December 7 to give you more time to choose and join a Medicare plan (page 13)

★ What's new (page 4)

★ What Medicare covers (page 31)

★ Your Medicare rights (page 105)

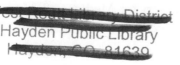
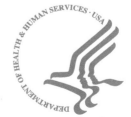

Welcome to Medicare & You 2012

This is an extraordinary time for health care in our Nation's history. We are working to make sure you have health care you can depend on—care that's focused on you, and is safe, effective, and timely, at a cost you can afford.

You may have heard about some of the exciting new changes Medicare has been making to help improve your health care—like more free preventive services and lower prescription drug costs.

There are some actions you can take right now to help keep yourself well. Medicare offers a number of preventive services to help keep you healthy and to find diseases early when treatments work best. Look at the checklist on the next page and take it with you on your next visit to your doctor or other health care provider. Use it to review and keep track of the preventive services that are right for you. Our goal is to help you achieve better health, better care, and lower costs.

One important new Medicare benefit—offered free of charge—is the Yearly "Wellness" visit. This is a chance for you and your doctor or other health care provider to review your health and talk about what you can do to stay as healthy as you can. To help you figure out what can help you stay well, your clinician may ask you to answer a short questionnaire called a Health Risk Assessment, as part of this visit. For more information about this and other important preventive services, visit www.medicare.gov/share-the-health.

This handbook is the best and official source of answers to your Medicare questions. We also have other helpful resources for you. Visit www.medicare.gov, or call 1-800-MEDICARE (1-800-633-4227) to get specific answers to your questions. You can also call your local State Health Insurance Assistance Program (SHIP). See pages 137–140 for the phone number. Or visit the Administration on Aging at www.aoa.gov.

Yours in good health,

Kathleen Sebelius

Secretary

U.S. Department of
Health and Human Services

Donald M. Berwick, MD

Administrator

Centers for Medicare & Medicaid
Services

Preventive Services Checklist

 Talk with your doctor or other health care provider about which of these services are right for you. As part of your Yearly "Wellness" visit, you may be asked to fill out a Health Risk Assessment to help you figure out what to work on to stay healthy. To learn more, visit www.medicare.gov.

Medicare-Covered Preventive Service	I Need (Yes/No)	Date Last Received	Next Date Medicare Covers This Service
"Welcome to Medicare" Preventive Visit (one-time)			
Yearly "Wellness" Visit			
Abdominal Aortic Aneurysm Screening			
Bone Mass Measurement			
Breast Cancer Screening (Mammogram)			
Cardiovascular Screenings			
Cervical and Vaginal Cancer Screening			
Colorectal Cancer Screenings			
Fecal Occult Blood Test			
Flexible Sigmoidoscopy			
Colonoscopy			
Barium Enema			
Diabetes Screenings			
Diabetes Self-Management Training			
Flu Shots			
Glaucoma Tests			
Hepatitis B Shots			
HIV Screening			
Medical Nutrition Therapy Services			
Pneumococcal Shot			
Prostate Cancer Screenings			
Tobacco Use Cessation Counseling (counseling for people with no sign of tobacco-related disease)			

For some services, you will need to wait a certain amount of time before getting the service again. See pages 37–53 for more information.

What's New and Important in 2012

New Dates to Change Plans   See pages 13, 78, and 85.

Starting this year, open enrollment begins and ends earlier—October 15–December 7, 2011.

New Special Enrollment Period   See pages 79 and 85.

You can switch to a Medicare Advantage Plan (like an HMO or PPO) or Medicare Prescription Drug Plan that has a 5-star rating at any time during the year.

Continued Help in the Prescription Drug Coverage Gap   See page 88.

If you reach the coverage gap in your Medicare prescription drug coverage, you will qualify for savings on brand-name and generic drugs.

Fighting Medicare Fraud   See page 117.

Find out what Medicare is doing and what you can do to protect against fraud, waste, and abuse.

Help with Long-term Care Costs   See page 123.

If you're still working, you may be able to enroll in a voluntary insurance program to help you pay for support services if you become disabled.

Better Coordination of Care   See pages 132–133.

Learn what Medicare and your health care providers are doing to better coordinate your health care and improve medical quality.

Ways to Manage Your Health Information Online   See page 135.

Learn about the new "Blue Button" on www.MyMedicare.gov that you can use to access your Medicare claims and other personal health information.

Medicare Health and Prescription Drug Plans

Visit www.medicare.gov/find-a-plan or call 1-800-MEDICARE (1-800-633-4227) to find plans in your area. TTY users should call 1-877-486-2048.

Where to Find Out What You Pay for Medicare (Part A and Part B). See the inside back cover.

The 2012 Medicare premium and deductible amounts weren't available at the time of printing. To get the most up-to-date cost information, visit www.medicare.gov or call 1-800-MEDICARE.

Blue words in the text are defined on pages 141–144.

Tools to Help You Find What You Need

Please keep this handbook for future reference. Information was correct when it was printed. Changes may occur after printing. Visit www.medicare.gov or call 1-800-MEDICARE (1-800-633-4227) to get the most current information. TTY users should call 1-877-486-2048.

Table of Contents	List of topics by section	Pages 6–8
Index	Alphabetical list of topics	Pages 9–12
Mini Tables of Contents	List of topics within each section	Pages 19, 31, 55, 97, 105, 121, 127
Blue words in the text	Blue words in the text are explained in the "Definitions" section	Pages 141–144
!	Highlights important information	Throughout handbook
🍎	Highlights preventive services	Pages 37–53
H	Highlights information related to Medicare Part A	Throughout handbook
👨‍⚕️	Highlights information related to Medicare Part B	Throughout handbook
H℞	Highlights information related to Medicare Part C	Throughout handbook
℞	Highlights information related to Medicare Part D	Throughout handbook

"Medicare & You" isn't a legal document. Official Medicare Program legal guidance is contained in the relevant statutes, regulations, and rulings.

Contents

Medicare & You 2012

Continued ⇒

Index

Note: The page number shown in **bold** provides the most detailed information.

Note: The page number shown in **bold** provides the most detailed information.

Note: The page number shown in **bold** provides the most detailed information.

Note: The page number shown in **bold** provides the most detailed information.

Important Enrollment Information

Coverage and Costs Change Yearly.

If you join a private Medicare health or prescription drug plan, your plan can change how much it costs and what it covers each year. Even if your plan's cost and coverage stay the same, your health or finances may have changed. Review your plan each year to make sure it will meet your needs for the following year. If you're satisfied that your current plan will meet your needs for next year, you don't need to do anything.

Fall Open Enrollment Period

Mark your calendar with these important dates! In most cases, this may be the one chance you have each year to make a change to your health and prescription drug coverage.

The fall Open Enrollment Period dates are earlier this year. The dates have changed to give you more time if you want to choose and join a Medicare health or prescription drug plan.

October 1– October 15, 2011	Compare your coverage with other available options to see if there's a better choice for you. See page 15.
October 15– December 7, 2011	**Open Enrollment Period. You can change your Medicare health or prescription drug coverage for 2012.** See pages 78 and 85 for other times when you can switch your coverage.
January 1, 2012	New coverage begins if you switched or joined a plan. New costs and benefit changes also begin if you kept your existing Medicare health or prescription drug coverage and your plan made changes.

Is your health or drug plan leaving Medicare? Health and prescription drug plans can decide not to participate in Medicare for the coming year. Your plan will send you a letter before the start of the Open Enrollment Period if it decides to leave Medicare or stop providing coverage in your area. See pages 106–107 for more information about your rights and options.

Medicare Basics

What is Medicare?

Medicare is health insurance for the following:

- People 65 or older
- People under 65 with certain disabilities
- People of any age with End-Stage Renal Disease (ESRD) (permanent kidney failure requiring dialysis or a kidney transplant)

The Different Parts of Medicare

The different parts of Medicare help cover specific services:

Medicare Part A (Hospital Insurance)

- Helps cover inpatient care in hospitals
- Helps cover skilled nursing facility, hospice, and home health care

See pages 32–35.

Medicare Part B (Medical Insurance)

- Helps cover doctors' and other health care providers' services, outpatient care, durable medical equipment, and home health care
- Helps cover some preventive services to help maintain your health and to keep certain illnesses from getting worse

See pages 36–53.

Medicare Part C (also known as Medicare Advantage)

Offers health plan options run by Medicare-approved private insurance companies. Medicare Advantage Plans are a way to get the benefits and services covered under Part A and Part B. Most Medicare Advantage Plans cover Medicare prescription drug coverage (Part D). Some Medicare Advantage Plans may include extra benefits for an extra cost.

See pages 70–81.

Medicare Part D (Medicare Prescription Drug Coverage)

- Helps cover the cost of prescription drugs
- May help lower your prescription drug costs and help protect against higher costs
- Run by Medicare-approved private insurance companies

See pages 84–94.

Your Medicare Coverage Choices at a Glance

There are two main ways to get your Medicare coverage: Original Medicare or a Medicare Advantage Plan. Use these steps to help you decide which way to get your coverage.

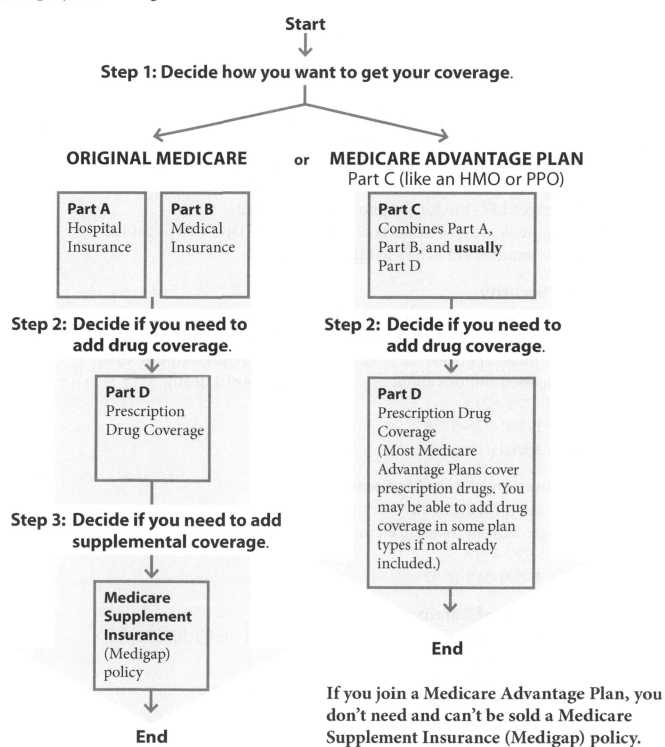

Start

Step 1: Decide how you want to get your coverage.

ORIGINAL MEDICARE   or   **MEDICARE ADVANTAGE PLAN**
Part C (like an HMO or PPO)

Part A
Hospital
Insurance

Part B
Medical
Insurance

Part C
Combines Part A,
Part B, and **usually**
Part D

Step 2: Decide if you need to add drug coverage.

Step 2: Decide if you need to add drug coverage.

Part D
Prescription
Drug Coverage

Part D
Prescription Drug
Coverage
(Most Medicare
Advantage Plans cover
prescription drugs. You
may be able to add drug
coverage in some plan
types if not already
included.)

Step 3: Decide if you need to add supplemental coverage.

**Medicare
Supplement
Insurance**
(Medigap)
policy

End

End

If you join a Medicare Advantage Plan, you don't need and can't be sold a Medicare Supplement Insurance (Medigap) policy.

See page 57 for more details.

Where to Get Your Medicare Questions Answered

1-800-MEDICARE (1-800-633-4227)
Get general or claims-specific Medicare information, help for people with limited income and resources, and important phone numbers. If you need help in a language other than English or Spanish, say "Agent" to talk to a customer service representative.
TTY 1-877-486-2048
www.medicare.gov

State Health Insurance Assistance Program (SHIP)
Get free personalized Medicare counseling on decisions about coverage; help with claims, billing, or appeals; and information on programs for people with limited income and resources.
See pages 137–140 for the phone number. Visit www.medicare.gov/contacts or call 1-800-MEDICARE to get the phone numbers of SHIPs in other states.

Social Security
Get a replacement Medicare card; change your address or name; get information about Part A and/or Part B eligibility, entitlement, and enrollment; apply for Extra Help with Medicare prescription drug costs; ask questions about premiums; and report a death.
1-800-772-1213
TTY 1-800-325-0778
www.socialsecurity.gov

Coordination of Benefits Contractor
Find out if Medicare or your other insurance pays first and to report changes in your insurance information.
1-800-999-1118
TTY 1-800-318-8782

Department of Defense
Get information about TRICARE for Life and the TRICARE Pharmacy Program.
1-866-773-0404 (TFL)
TTY 1-866-773-0405
1-877-363-1303 (Pharmacy)
TTY 1-877-540-6261
www.tricare.mil/mybenefit

Department of Health and Human Services

Office for Civil Rights

If you think you were discriminated against or if your health information privacy rights were violated.

1-800-368-1019

TTY 1-800-537-7697

www.hhs.gov/ocr

Department of Veterans Affairs

If you're a veteran or have served in the U.S. military.

1-800-827-1000

TTY 1-800-829-4833

www.va.gov

Office of Personnel Management

Get information about the Federal Employee Health Benefits Program for current and retired Federal employees.

1-888-767-6738

TTY 1-800-878-5707

www.opm.gov/insure

Railroad Retirement Board (RRB)

If you have benefits from the RRB, call them to change your address or name, check eligibility, enroll in Medicare, replace your Medicare card, or report a death.

Local RRB office or 1-877-772-5772

www.rrb.gov

Quality Improvement Organization (QIO)

Ask questions or report complaints about the quality of care for a Medicare-covered service or if you think Medicare coverage for your service is ending too soon. Visit www.medicare.gov/contacts or call 1-800-MEDICARE to get the phone number for your QIO.

Notes

Signing Up for Medicare Part A and Part B

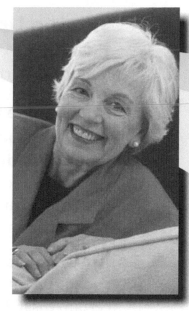

Section 1 includes information about the following:

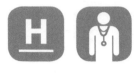

Signing Up for Part A and Part B

This section explains how and when to sign up and if you should wait to get Part B.

Some People Get Part A and Part B Automatically

Are you already getting benefits from Social Security or the Railroad Retirement Board (RRB)? If you are, in most cases, you will automatically get Part A and Part B starting the first day of the month you turn 65. If your birthday is on the first day of the month, Part A and Part B will start the first day of the prior month.

Are you under 65 and disabled? If so, you automatically get Part A and Part B after you get disability benefits from Social Security or certain disability benefits from the RRB for 24 months.

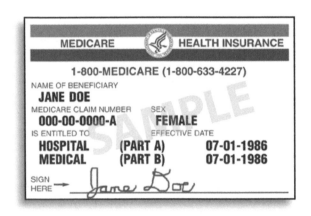

If you're automatically enrolled, you will get your red, white, and blue Medicare card in the mail 3 months before your 65th birthday or your 25th month of disability. If you don't want Part B, follow the instructions that come with the card, and send the card back. If you keep the card, you keep Part B and will pay Part B premiums. See page 24 for help deciding if you need to sign up for Part B.

Do you have ALS (Amyotrophic Lateral Sclerosis, also called Lou Gehrig's disease)? If you do, you automatically get Part A and Part B the month your disability benefits begin.

Do you live in Puerto Rico and get benefits from Social Security or the RRB? If so, you will automatically get Part A. If you want Part B, you will need to sign up for it. Contact your local Social Security office or RRB for more information.

Do you have Part A and TRICARE (insurance for active duty military or retirees and their families)? If you do, you must have Part B to keep your TRICARE coverage. See page 25.

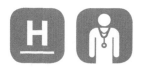

Signing Up for Part A and Part B (continued)

Some People Need to Sign Up for Part A and Part B

Are you close to 65, but not getting Social Security or Railroad Retirement Board (RRB) benefits? If you aren't getting Social Security or RRB benefits (for example, because you're still working) and you want Part A or Part B, **you will need to sign up** (even if you're eligible to get Part A premium-free). If you're not eligible for premium-free Part A, you can buy Part A and Part B.

Contact Social Security 3 months before you turn 65. If you worked for a railroad, contact the RRB to sign up.

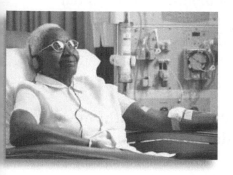

Do you have End-Stage Renal Disease (ESRD)? If you do, visit your local Social Security office, or call Social Security at 1-800-772-1213 to sign up for Part A and Part B. TTY users should call 1-800-325-0778. For more information, visit www.medicare.gov/publications to view the booklet "Medicare Coverage of Kidney Dialysis and Kidney Transplant Services." You can also call 1-800-MEDICARE (1-800-633-4227) to find out if a copy can be mailed to you. TTY users should call 1-877-486-2048.

Call Social Security at 1-800-772-1213 for more information about your Medicare eligibility, and to sign up for Part A and/or Part B. If you're 65 or older, you can also apply for premium-free Part A and Part B (for which you pay a monthly premium) at www.socialsecurity.gov/retirement. The whole process can take less than 10 minutes. If you get RRB benefits, call the RRB at 1-877-772-5772.

For general information about enrolling, visit www.medicare.gov/MedicareEligibility. You can also get free, personalized health insurance counseling from your State Health Insurance Assistance Program (SHIP). See pages 137–140 for the phone number.

Blue words in the text are defined on pages 141–144.

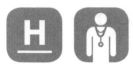

When Can You Sign Up?

Initial Enrollment Period

You can sign up when you're first eligible for Part A and/or Part B (for which you pay monthly premiums) during your Initial Enrollment Period. For example, if you're eligible when you turn 65, you can sign up during the 7-month period that begins 3 months before the month you turn 65, includes the month you turn 65, and ends 3 months after the month you turn 65.

3 months before the month you turn **65**	**2** months before the month you turn **65**	**1** month before the month you turn **65**	The month you turn **65**	**1** month after you turn **65**	**2** months after you turn **65**	**3** months after you turn **65**
Sign up early to avoid a delay in coverage. To get Part A and/or Part B the month you turn 65, you must sign up during the first 3 months before the month you turn 65.			If you wait until the last 4 months of your Initial Enrollment Period to sign up for Part A and/or Part B, your coverage will be delayed. See chart below.			

Note:

If you're automatically enrolled, these enrollment periods don't apply to you.

If you sign up for Part A and/or Part B during the first 3 months of your Initial Enrollment Period, your coverage start date will depend on your birthday:

- If your birthday **isn't** on the first day of the month, your Part B coverage starts the first day of your birthday month. For example, Mr. Green's 65th birthday is July 20, 2012. If he enrolls in April, May, or June, his coverage will start on July 1, 2012.
- If your birthday **is** on the first day of the month, your coverage will start the first day of the prior month. For example, Mr. Kim's 65th birthday is July 1, 2012. If he enrolls in March, April, or May, his coverage will start on June 1, 2012. To read the chart above correctly, use the month **before** your birthday as "the month you turn 65."

If you enroll in Part A and/or Part B the month you turn 65 or during the last 3 months of your Initial Enrollment Period, your start date will be delayed:

If you enroll in this month of your initial enrollment period:	Your coverage starts:
The month you turn 65	1 month after enrollment
1 month after you turn 65	2 months after enrollment
2 months after you turn 65	3 months after enrollment
3 months after you turn 65	3 months after enrollment

When Can You Sign Up? (continued)

General Enrollment Period

If you didn't sign up for Part A and/or Part B (for which you pay monthly premiums) when you were first eligible, you can sign up between January 1–March 31 each year. Your coverage will begin July 1. You may have to pay a higher premium for late enrollment. See pages 28 and 30.

If you sign up during these months:	Your coverage will begin on:
January	
February	July 1
March	

Special Enrollment Period

If you didn't sign up for Part A and/or Part B (for which you pay monthly premiums) when you were first eligible because you're covered under a group health plan based on **current employment**, you can sign up for Part A and/or Part B as follows:

Anytime that you or your spouse (or family member if you're disabled) is working, and you're covered by a group health plan through the employer or union based on that work	Or	**During the 8-month period that begins the month after the employment ends or the group health plan insurance based on current employment ends, whichever happens first**

Usually, you don't pay a late enrollment penalty if you sign up during a Special Enrollment Period. This Special Enrollment Period doesn't apply to people with End-Stage Renal Disease (ESRD). See page 21. You may also qualify for a Special Enrollment Period if you're a volunteer serving in a foreign country.

Note: COBRA and retiree health plans aren't considered coverage based on current employment. You're not eligible for a Special Enrollment Period when that coverage ends. To avoid paying a higher premium, make sure you sign up for Medicare when you're first eligible.

Blue words in the text are defined on pages 141–144.

Medicare Supplement Insurance (Medigap) Open Enrollment Period

Medicare Supplement Insurance (Medigap) policies, sold by private insurance companies, help pay some of the health care costs that Medicare doesn't cover. You have a 6-month Medigap Open Enrollment Period which starts the first month you're 65 **and** enrolled in Part B. This period gives you a guaranteed right to buy any Medigap policy sold in your state regardless of your health status. Once this period starts, it can't be delayed or replaced. See pages 66–69.

Blue words in the text are defined on pages 141–144.

To learn more details about enrollment periods, visit www.medicare.gov/publications to view the fact sheet "Understanding Medicare Enrollment Periods." You can also call 1-800-MEDICARE (1-800-633-4227) to find out if a copy can be mailed to you. TTY users should call 1-877-486-2048.

Should You Get Part B?

The following information can help you decide if you want to sign up for Part B.

Employer or Union Coverage—If you or your spouse (or family member if you're disabled) **is still working** and you have health coverage through that employer (including the Federal Employee Health Benefits Program) or union, contact your employer or union benefits administrator to find out how your coverage works with Medicare. It may be to your advantage to delay Part B enrollment.

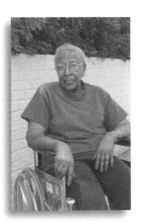

You can sign up for Part B any time you have current employer health coverage. COBRA and retiree health coverage don't count as current employer coverage.

Once the employment ends, three things happen:

1. You have 8 months to sign up for Part B without a penalty. This period will run whether or not you choose COBRA. **If you choose COBRA, don't wait until your COBRA ends to enroll in Part B.** If you don't enroll in Part B during the 8 months, you may have to pay a penalty. You won't be able to enroll until the next General Enrollment Period and you will have to wait before your coverage begins. See page 23.

Should You Get Part B? (continued)

2. You may be able to get COBRA coverage, which continues your health insurance through the employer's plan (in most cases for only 18 months) and probably at a higher cost to you.

   — If you already have COBRA coverage when you enroll in Medicare, your COBRA will probably end.

   — If you become eligible for COBRA coverage after you're already enrolled in Medicare, you must be allowed to take the COBRA coverage. It will always be secondary to Medicare (unless you have End-Stage Renal Disease (ESRD)).

3. When you sign up for Part B, your Medigap Open Enrollment Period begins. See page 68.

TRICARE—If you have Part A and TRICARE (insurance for active-duty military or retirees and their families), **you must have Part B to keep your TRICARE coverage.** However, if you're an active-duty service member, or the spouse or dependent child of an active-duty service member, the following applies to you:

- You don't have to enroll in Part B to keep your TRICARE coverage while the service member is on active duty.

- Before the active-duty service member retires, you must enroll in Part B to keep TRICARE without a break in coverage.

- You can get Part B during a special enrollment period if you have Medicare because you're 65 or older, or you're disabled.

- You don't need to re-enroll in TRICARE each year. Your coverage will continue as long as you have Part B.

How Other Insurance Works with Medicare

When you have other insurance (like employer group health coverage), there are rules that decide whether Medicare or your other insurance pays first. The insurance that pays first is called the "**primary payer.**" The one that pays second is called the "**secondary payer.**"

Use this chart to see who pays first.

If you have **retiree** insurance (insurance from former employment)…	Medicare pays first.
If you're 65 or older, have group health plan coverage based on your or your spouse's **current** employment, and the employer has **20 or more employees**…	Your group health plan pays first.
If you're 65 or older, have group health plan coverage based on your or your spouse's **current** employment, and the employer has **less than 20 employees**…	Medicare pays first.
If you're under 65 and disabled, have group health plan coverage based on your or a family member's **current** employment, and the employer has **100 or more employees**…	Your group health plan pays first.
If you're under 65 and disabled, have group health plan coverage based on your or a family member's **current** employment, and the employer has **less than 100 employees**…	Medicare pays first.
If you have Medicare because of End-Stage Renal Disease (ESRD)…	Your group health plan will pay first for the first 30 months after you become eligible to enroll in Medicare. Medicare will pay first after this 30-month period.

 Note: In some cases, your employer may join with other employers or unions to form a multiple employer plan. If this happens, only one of the employers or unions in the multiple employer plan has to have the required number of employees for group health plan to pay first.

How Other Insurance Works with Medicare (continued)

Here are some important facts to remember:

- The insurance that pays first (primary payer) pays up to the limits of its coverage.
- The one that pays second (secondary payer) only pays if there are costs the primary insurer didn't cover.
- The secondary payer (which may be Medicare) may not pay all of the uncovered costs.
- If your employer insurance is the secondary payer, you may need to enroll in Part B before your insurance will pay.

These types of insurance usually pay first for services related to each type:

- No-fault insurance (including automobile insurance)
- Liability (including automobile insurance)
- Black lung benefits
- Workers' compensation

Medicaid and TRICARE never pay first for services that are covered by Medicare. They only pay after Medicare, employer group health plans, and/or Medicare Supplement Insurance have paid.

For more information, visit www.medicare.gov/publications to view the booklet "Medicare and Other Health Benefits: Your Guide to Who Pays First." You can also call 1-800-MEDICARE (1-800-633-4227) to find out if a copy can be mailed to you. TTY users should call 1-877-486-2048.

Blue words in the text are defined on pages 141–144.

If you have other insurance, tell your doctor, hospital, and pharmacy. If you have questions about who pays first, or you need to update your other insurance information, call Medicare's Coordination of Benefits Contractor at 1-800-999-1118. TTY users should call 1-800-318-8782. You can also contact your employer or union benefits administrator. You may need to give your Medicare number to your other insurers so your bills are paid correctly and on time.

How Much Does Part A Coverage Cost?

You usually don't pay a monthly premium for Part A coverage if you or your spouse paid Medicare taxes while working.

If you aren't eligible for premium-free Part A, you may be able to buy Part A if you meet one of the following conditions:

- You're 65 or older, and you have (or are enrolling in) Part B and meet the citizenship and residency requirements.
- You're under 65, disabled, and your premium-free Part A coverage ended because you returned to work. (If you're under 65 and disabled, you can continue to get premium-free Part A for up to 8 1/2 years after you return to work.)

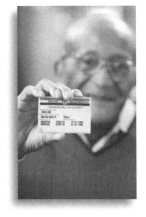

Note: In 2011, people who had to buy Part A paid up to $450 each month. Visit www.medicare.gov or call 1-800-MEDICARE (1-800-633-4227) to find out the amount for 2012. TTY users should call 1-877-486-2048.

In most cases, if you choose to **buy** Part A, you must also have Part B and pay monthly premiums for both. If you have limited income and resources, your state may help you pay for Part A and/or Part B. See page 102. Call Social Security at 1-800-772-1213 for more information about the Part A premium. TTY users should call 1-800-325-0778.

Part A Late Enrollment Penalty

If you aren't eligible for premium-free Part A, and you don't buy it when you're first eligible, your monthly premium may go up 10%. You will have to pay the higher premium for twice the number of years you could have had Part A, but didn't sign-up. For example, if you were eligible for Part A for 2 years but didn't sign-up, you will have to pay the higher premium for 4 years. Usually, you don't have to pay a penalty if you meet certain conditions that allow you to sign up for Part A during a Special Enrollment Period. See page 23.

How Much Does Part B Coverage Cost?

You pay the Part B premium each month. Most people will pay up to the standard premium amount. However, if your modified adjusted gross income as reported on your IRS tax return from 2 years ago (the most recent tax return information provided to Social Security by the IRS) is above a certain amount, you may pay more.

Your modified adjusted gross income is your adjusted gross income plus your tax exempt interest income. Each year, Social Security will notify you if you have to pay more than the standard premium. The amount you pay can change each year depending on your income. If you have to pay a higher amount for your Part B premium and you disagree (for example, if your income goes down), call Social Security at 1-800-772-1213. TTY users should call 1-800-325-0778. If you get benefits from RRB, you should also contact Social Security.

Visit www.socialsecurity.gov/pubs/10536.pdf to view the fact sheet "Medicare Premiums: Rules for Higher-Income Beneficiaries."

The standard Part B premium in 2011 was $115.40. Visit www.medicare.gov or call 1-800 MEDICARE (1-800-633-4227) to find out the amount for 2012. TTY users should call 1-877-486-2048.

Blue words in the text are defined on pages 141–144.

How Much Does Part B Coverage Cost? (continued)

Ways to Pay

If you get Social Security, RRB, or Civil Service benefits, your Part B premium will get deducted from your benefit payment. If you don't get these benefit payments and choose to sign up for Part B, you will get a bill. If you choose to buy Part A, you will always get a bill for your premium. You can mail your premium payments to the Medicare Premium Collection Center, P.O. Box 790355, St. Louis, Missouri 63179-0355. If you get a bill from the RRB, mail your premium payments to RRB, Medicare Premium Payments, P.O. Box 9024, St. Louis, Missouri 63197-9024.

Part B Late Enrollment Penalty

If you don't sign up for Part B when you're first eligible, you may have to pay a late enrollment penalty for as long as you have Medicare. Your monthly premium for Part B may go up 10% for each full 12-month period that you could have had Part B, but didn't sign up for it. Usually, you don't pay a late enrollment penalty if you meet certain conditions that allow you to sign up for Part B during a special enrollment period. See page 23.

Example: Mr. Smith's initial enrollment period ended September 30, 2008. He waited to sign up for Part B until the General Enrollment Period in March 2011. His Part B premium penalty is 20%. (While Mr. Smith waited a total of 30 months to sign up, this included only two full 12-month periods.)

If you have limited income and resources, see page 97 for information about help paying your Medicare premiums.

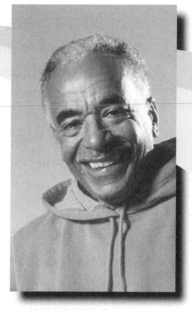

What Medicare Part A and Part B Cover

Section 2 includes information about the following:

What Services Does Medicare Cover?

Medicare covers certain medical services and supplies in hospitals, doctors' offices, and other health care settings. Services are either covered under Part A or Part B. If you have both Part A and Part B, you can get all of the Medicare-covered services listed in this section, whether you have Original Medicare or a Medicare health plan.

- See pages 33–35 for the Part A-covered services list.
- See pages 37–53 for the Part B-covered services list.

What Does Part A (Hospital Insurance) Cover?

Part A helps cover the following:

- Inpatient care in hospitals
- Inpatient care in a skilled nursing facility (not custodial or long-term care)
- Hospice care services
- Home health care services
- Inpatient care in a Religious Nonmedical Health Care Institution

You can find out if you have Part A by looking at your Medicare card. If you have Original Medicare, you will use this card to get your Medicare-covered services. If you join a Medicare health plan, you must use the card from the plan to get your Medicare-covered services.

What You Pay for Part A-Covered Services

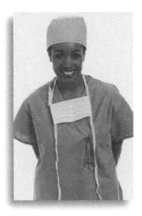

Copayments, coinsurance, and deductibles may apply for each service in the list on the next three pages. Visit www.medicare.gov or call 1-800-MEDICARE (1-800-633-4227) to get specific cost information. TTY users should call 1-877-486-2048.

If you're in a Medicare health plan or have other insurance (like a Medicare Supplement Insurance (Medigap) policy, or employer or union coverage), your costs may be different. Contact the plans you're interested in to find out about the costs, or visit the Medicare Plan Finder at www.medicare.gov/find-a-plan.

Part A-Covered Services

Blood

In most cases, the hospital gets blood from a blood bank at no charge, and you won't have to pay for it or replace it. If the hospital has to buy blood for you, you must either pay the hospital costs for the first 3 units of blood you get in a calendar year or have the blood donated by you or someone else.

Home Health Services

Medicare covers medically-necessary part-time or intermittent skilled nursing care, and/or physical therapy, speech-language pathology services, and/or services for people with a continuing need for occupational therapy. A doctor enrolled in Medicare, or certain health care providers who work with the doctor, must see you face-to-face before the doctor can certify that you need home health services. That doctor must order your care, and a Medicare-certified home health agency must provide it. Home health services may also include medical social services, part-time or intermittent home health aide services, and medical supplies for use at home. You must be homebound, which means leaving home is a major effort.

- You pay nothing for covered home health care services.
- You pay 20% of the Medicare-approved amount for durable medical equipment. See page 42.

Hospice Care

To qualify for hospice care, your doctor must certify that you're terminally ill and have 6 months or less to live. If you're already getting hospice care, a hospice doctor or nurse practitioner will need to see you about 6 months after you enter hospice to certify that you're still terminally ill. Coverage includes drugs for pain relief and symptom management; medical, nursing, and social services; certain durable medical equipment and other covered services as well as services Medicare usually doesn't cover, such as spiritual and grief counseling. A Medicare-approved hospice usually gives hospice care in your home or other facility where you live such as a nursing home.

Blue words in the text are defined on pages 141–144.

H

Part A-Covered Services

Hospice Care (continued)

Hospice care doesn't pay for your stay in a facility (room and board) unless the hospice medical team determines that you need short-term inpatient stays for pain and symptom management that can't be addressed at home. These stays must be in a Medicare-approved facility, such as a hospice facility, hospital, or skilled nursing facility which contracts with the hospice. Medicare also covers inpatient respite care which is care you get in a Medicare-approved facility so that your usual caregiver can rest. You can stay up to 5 days each time you get respite care. Medicare will pay for covered services for health problems that aren't related to your terminal illness. You can continue to get hospice care as long as the hospice medical director or hospice doctor recertifies that you're terminally ill.

- You pay nothing for hospice care.
- You pay a copayment of up to $5 per prescription for outpatient prescription drugs for pain and symptom management.
- You pay 5% of the Medicare-approved amount for inpatient respite care.

Hospital Care (Inpatient)

Medicare covers semi-private rooms, meals, general nursing, and drugs as part of your inpatient treatment, and other hospital services and supplies. This includes care you get in acute care hospitals, critical access hospitals, inpatient rehabilitation facilities, long-term care hospitals, inpatient care as part of a qualifying clinical research study, and mental health care. This **doesn't** include private-duty nursing, a television or phone in your room (if there is a separate charge for these items), or personal care items like razors or slipper socks. It also doesn't include a private room, unless medically necessary. If you have Part B, it covers the doctor's services you get while you're in a hospital.

Blue words in the text are defined on pages 141–144.

- You pay a deductible and no copayment for days 1–60 each benefit period.
- You pay a copayment for days 61–90 each benefit period.
- You pay a copayment per "lifetime reserve day" after day 90 each benefit period (up to 60 days over your lifetime).
- You pay all costs for each day after the lifetime reserve days.
- Inpatient mental health care in a psychiatric hospital is limited to 190 days in a lifetime.

Part A-Covered Services

Hospital Care (Inpatient) (continued)

Note: Staying overnight in a hospital doesn't always mean you're an inpatient. You're considered an inpatient the day a doctor formally admits you to a hospital with a doctor's order. Always ask if you're an inpatient or an outpatient since it **affects what you pay and whether you will qualify for Part A coverage in a** skilled nursing facility. For more information, visit www.medicare.gov/publications to view the fact sheet "Are You a Hospital Inpatient or Outpatient? If You Have Medicare—Ask!" You can also call 1-800-MEDICARE (1-800-633-4227) to find out if a copy can be mailed to you. TTY users should call 1-877-486-2048.

Religious Nonmedical Health Care Institution (Inpatient care)

Medicare will only cover the non-medical, non-religious health care items and services (like room and board) in this type of facility if you qualify for hospital or skilled nursing facility care, but your medical care isn't in agreement with your religious beliefs. Non-medical items and services, like wound dressings or use of a simple walker during your stay, don't require a doctor's order or prescription. Medicare doesn't cover the religious portion of care.

Skilled Nursing Facility Care

Medicare covers semi-private rooms, meals, skilled nursing and rehabilitative services, and other services and supplies that are medically necessary after a **3-day minimum medically-necessary inpatient hospital stay** for a related illness or injury. An inpatient hospital stay begins the day you're formally admitted with a doctor's order and doesn't include the day you're discharged. To qualify for care in a skilled nursing facility, your doctor must certify that you need daily skilled care like intravenous injections or physical therapy. Medicare **doesn't** cover long-term care or custodial care.

- You pay nothing for the first 20 days each benefit period.
- You pay a coinsurance per day for days 21–100 each benefit period.
- You pay all costs for each day after day 100 in a benefit period.

Note: Visit www.medicare.gov or call 1-800-MEDICARE to find out what you pay for inpatient hospital stays and skilled nursing facility care in 2012.

What Does Part B (Medical Insurance) Cover?

Part B helps cover medically-necessary services like doctors' services, outpatient care, home health services, durable medical equipment, and other medical services. Part B also covers many preventive services. You can find out if you have Part B by looking at your Medicare card.

Pages 37–53 include a list of common Part B-covered services and general descriptions. Medicare may cover some services and tests more often than the timeframes listed if needed to diagnose a condition. To find out if Medicare covers a service not on this list, visit www.medicare.gov/coverage or call 1-800-MEDICARE (1-800-633-4227). TTY users should call 1-877-486-2048. For more details about Medicare-covered services, visit www.medicare.gov/publications to view the booklet "Your Medicare Benefits."

You will see this apple next to the preventive services on pages 37–53. Use the preventive services checklist on page 3 to ask your doctor or other health care provider which preventive services you should get.

What You Pay for Part B-Covered Services

The alphabetical list on the following pages gives general information about what you pay if you have Original Medicare and see doctors or other health care providers who accept assignment. You will pay more for doctors or providers who don't accept assignment. **If you're in a Medicare Advantage Plan (like an HMO or PPO) or have other insurance, your costs may be different. Contact your plan or benefits administrator directly to find out about the costs.**

Under Original Medicare, if the Part B deductible applies you must pay all costs until you meet the yearly Part B deductible before Medicare begins to pay its share. Then, after your deductible is met, you typically pay 20% of the Medicare-approved amount of the service, if the doctor or other health care provider accepts assignment. There is no yearly limit for what you pay out-of-pocket. Visit www.medicare.gov or call 1-800-MEDICARE to get specific cost information.

You pay nothing for most preventive services if you get the services from a doctor or other health care provider who accepts assignment. However, for some preventive services, you may have to pay a deductible, coinsurance, or both.

Note: See page 62 for more information about assignment.

Part B-Covered Services

Abdominal Aortic Aneurysm Screening

Medicare covers a one-time screening abdominal aortic aneurysm ultrasound for people at risk. You must get a referral for it as part of your one-time "Welcome to Medicare" preventive visit. See page 53. You pay nothing for the screening if the doctor or other health care provider accepts assignment.

Ambulance Services

Medicare covers ground ambulance transportation when you need to be transported to a hospital or skilled nursing facility for medically-necessary services, and transportation in any other vehicle could endanger your health. Medicare may pay for emergency ambulance transportation in an airplane or helicopter to a hospital if you need immediate and rapid ambulance transportation that ground transportation can't provide.

In some cases, Medicare may pay for limited non-emergency ambulance transportation if you have orders from your doctor saying that ambulance transportation is medically necessary. Medicare will only cover ambulance services to the nearest appropriate medical facility that's able to give you the care you need. You pay 20% of the Medicare-approved amount, and the Part B deductible applies.

Ambulatory Surgical Centers

Medicare covers the facility fees for approved surgical procedures in an ambulatory surgical center (facility where surgical procedures are performed, and the patient is released within 24 hours). Except for certain preventive services (for which you pay nothing), you pay 20% of the Medicare-approved amount to both the ambulatory surgical center and the doctor who treats you, and the Part B deductible applies. You pay all facility fees for procedures Medicare doesn't allow in ambulatory surgical centers.

Part B-Covered Services

Blood

In most cases, the provider gets blood from a blood bank at no charge, and you won't have to pay for it or replace it. However, you will pay a copayment for the blood processing and handling services for every unit of blood you get, and the Part B deductible applies. If the provider has to buy blood for you, you must either pay the provider costs for the first 3 units of blood you get in a calendar year or have the blood donated by you or someone else.

Bone Mass Measurement (Bone Density)

This test helps to see if you're at risk for broken bones. It's covered once every 24 months (more often if medically necessary) for people who have certain medical conditions or meet certain criteria. You pay nothing for this test if the doctor or other health care provider accepts assignment.

Breast Cancer Screening (Mammograms)

Medicare covers screening mammograms to check for breast cancer once every 12 months for all women with Medicare 40 and older. Medicare covers one baseline mammogram for women between 35–39. You pay nothing for the test if the doctor or other health care provider accepts assignment.

Cardiac Rehabilitation

Medicare covers comprehensive programs that include exercise, education, and counseling for patients who meet certain conditions. Medicare also covers intensive cardiac rehabilitation programs that are typically more rigorous or more intense than regular cardiac rehabilitation programs. You pay 20% of the Medicare-approved amount if you get the services in a doctor's office. In a hospital outpatient setting, you also pay the hospital a copayment. The Part B deductible applies.

Part B-Covered Services

Cardiovascular Screenings

These screenings include blood tests that help detect conditions that may lead to a heart attack or stroke. Medicare covers these screening tests every 5 years to test your cholesterol, lipid, and triglyceride levels. You pay nothing for the tests, but you generally have to pay 20% of the Medicare-approved amount for the doctor's visit.

Cervical and Vaginal Cancer Screening

Medicare covers Pap tests and pelvic exams to check for cervical and vaginal cancers. As part of the exam, Medicare also covers a clinical breast exam to check for breast cancer. Medicare covers these screening tests once every 24 months. Medicare covers these screening tests once every 12 months if you're at high risk for cervical or vaginal cancer or if you're of child-bearing age and had an abnormal Pap test in the past 36 months. You pay nothing for the Pap lab test, Pap test specimen collection, and pelvic and breast exams if the doctor or other health care provider accepts assignment.

Chemotherapy

Medicare covers chemotherapy in a doctor's office, freestanding clinic, or hospital outpatient setting for people with cancer. For chemotherapy given in a doctor's office or freestanding clinic, you pay 20% of the Medicare-approved amount. If you get chemotherapy in a hospital outpatient setting, you pay a copayment for the treatment. For chemotherapy in a hospital inpatient setting covered under Part A, see Hospital Care (Inpatient) on page 34.

Chiropractic Services (limited)

Medicare covers these services to help correct a subluxation (when one or more of the bones of your spine move out of position) using manipulation of the spine. You pay 20% of the Medicare-approved amount, and the Part B deductible applies.

Note: You pay all costs for any other services or tests ordered by a chiropractor (including X-rays or massage therapy).

Part B-Covered Services

Clinical Research Studies

Clinical research studies test how well different types of medical care work and if they are safe. Medicare covers some costs, like office visits and tests, in qualifying clinical research studies. You pay 20% of the Medicare-approved amount, and the Part B deductible applies.
Note: If you're in a Medicare Advantage Plan (like an HMO or PPO), some costs may be covered by your plan.

Colorectal Cancer Screenings

Medicare covers these screenings to help find precancerous growths or find cancer early, when treatment is most effective. One or more of the following tests may be covered. Talk to your doctor or other health care provider.

- Fecal Occult Blood Test—This test is covered once every 12 months if you're 50 or older. You pay nothing for the test.
- Flexible Sigmoidoscopy—This test is generally covered once every 48 months if you're 50 or older, or 120 months after a previous screening colonoscopy for those not at high risk. You pay nothing for this test if the doctor or other health care provider accepts assignment.
- Colonoscopy—This test is generally covered once every 120 months (high risk every 24 months) or 48 months after a previous flexible sigmoidoscopy. No minimum age. You pay nothing for this test if the doctor or other health care provider accepts assignment.
- Barium Enema—This test is generally covered once every 48 months if you're 50 or older (high risk every 24 months) when used instead of a sigmoidoscopy or colonoscopy. You pay 20% of the Medicare-approved amount for the doctor services. In a hospital outpatient setting, you also pay the hospital a copayment.

Defibrillator (Implantable Automatic)

Medicare covers these devices for some people diagnosed with heart failure. If the surgery takes place in an outpatient setting, you pay 20% of the Medicare-approved amount for the doctor's services. If you get the device as a hospital outpatient, you also pay the hospital a copayment, but no more than the Part A hospital stay deductible. The Part B deductible applies. Surgeries to implant defibrillators in a hospital inpatient setting are covered under Part A. See Hospital Care (Inpatient) on page 34.

Part B-Covered Services

Diabetes Screenings

Medicare covers these screenings if you have any of the following risk factors: high blood pressure (hypertension), history of abnormal cholesterol and triglyceride levels (dyslipidemia), obesity, or a history of high blood glucose (blood sugar). Tests may also be covered if you meet other requirements, like being overweight or having a family history of diabetes.

Based on the results of these tests, you may be eligible for up to two diabetes screenings every year. You pay nothing for the test if your doctor or other health care provider accepts assignment.

Diabetes Self-Management Training

Medicare covers a program to help people cope with and manage diabetes. The program may include tips for eating healthy, being active, monitoring blood sugar, taking medication, and reducing risks. You must have diabetes and a written order from your doctor or other health care provider. You pay 20% of the Medicare-approved amount, and the Part B deductible applies.

Diabetes Supplies

Medicare covers blood sugar testing monitors, blood sugar test strips, lancet devices and lancets, blood sugar control solutions, and therapeutic shoes (in some cases). Medicare only covers insulin if used with an external insulin pump. You pay 20% of the Medicare-approved amount, and the Part B deductible applies.

Note: Medicare prescription drug coverage (Part D) may cover insulin and certain medical supplies used to inject insulin, such as syringes, and some oral diabetic drugs.

Doctor and Other Health Care Provider Services

Medicare covers doctor services that are medically necessary (includes outpatient and some doctor services you get when you're a hospital inpatient) or covered preventive services. Medicare also covers services provided by other health care providers, such as physician assistants, nurse practitioners, social workers, physical therapists, and psychologists. Except for certain preventive services (for which you pay nothing), you pay 20% of the Medicare-approved amount, and the Part B deductible applies.

Part B-Covered Services

Durable Medical Equipment (like walkers)

Medicare covers items such as oxygen equipment and supplies, wheelchairs, walkers, and hospital beds ordered by a doctor or other health care provider enrolled in Medicare for use in the home. Some items must be rented. You pay 20% of the Medicare-approved amount, and the Part B deductible applies. **In all areas of the country, you must get your covered equipment or supplies and replacement or repair services from a Medicare-approved supplier for Medicare to pay.**

For more information, visit www.medicare.gov/publications to view the booklet "Medicare Coverage of Durable Medical Equipment and Other Devices."

In some areas of the country if you need certain items, you must use specific suppliers, or Medicare won't pay for the item and you likely will pay full price. This program will help save you and Medicare money; ensure you get quality equipment, supplies, and services; and help limit fraud and abuse. It's important to see if you're affected by this program to ensure Medicare payment and avoid any disruption of service.

This program is effective in certain areas in the following states: California, Florida, Indiana, Kansas, Kentucky, Missouri, North Carolina, Ohio, Pennsylvania, South Carolina, and Texas. If you currently live in or visit one of these areas and are renting or need certain durable medical equipment or supplies, do any of the following to get answers to your questions about what's covered or about suppliers:

- Visit www.medicare.gov/supplier. Medicare-approved suppliers are listed. The specific suppliers you need to use for this new program have an orange star next to their names.
- Call 1-800-MEDICARE (1-800-633-4227). TTY users should call 1-877-486-2048.
- Call your State Health Insurance Assistance Program (SHIP). See pages 137–140 for the phone number.

The program will expand to 91 additional areas around the country in 2013. Medicare will provide more information before changes occur in those areas.

Part B-Covered Services

EKG (Electrocardiogram) Screening

Medicare covers a one-time screening EKG if ordered by your doctor or other health care provider as part of your one-time "Welcome to Medicare" preventive visit. See page 53. You pay 20% of the Medicare-approved amount, and the Part B deductible applies. An EKG is also covered as a diagnostic test. See page 50. If you have the test at a hospital or a hospital owned clinic, you also pay the hospital a copayment.

Emergency Department Services

These services are covered when you have an injury, a sudden illness, or an illness that quickly gets much worse. You pay a specified copayment for the hospital emergency department visit, and you pay 20% of the Medicare-approved amount for the doctor's or other health care provider's services. The Part B deductible applies.

Eyeglasses (limited)

Medicare covers one pair of eyeglasses with standard frames (or one set of contact lenses) after cataract surgery that implants an intraocular lens. You pay 20% of the Medicare-approved amount, and the Part B deductible applies.

Federally-Qualified Health Center Services

Medicare covers many outpatient primary care and preventive services you get through certain community-based organizations. Generally, you pay 20% of the Medicare-approved amount. You pay nothing for most preventive services.

Flu Shots

Medicare generally covers flu shots once per flu season in the fall or winter. You pay nothing for getting the flu shot if the doctor or other health care provider accepts assignment for giving the shot.

Foot Exams and Treatment

Medicare covers foot exams and treatment if you have diabetes-related nerve damage and/or meet certain conditions. You pay 20% of the Medicare-approved amount, and the Part B deductible applies. In a hospital outpatient setting, you also pay the hospital a copayment.

Part B-Covered Services

Glaucoma Tests

These tests are covered once every 12 months for people at high risk for the eye disease glaucoma. You're at high risk if you have diabetes, a family history of glaucoma, are African-American and 50 or older, or are Hispanic and 65 or older. An eye doctor who is legally allowed by the state must do the tests. You pay 20% of the Medicare-approved amount, and the Part B deductible applies for the doctor's visit. In a hospital outpatient setting, you also pay the hospital a copayment.

Hearing and Balance Exams

Medicare covers these exams if your doctor or other health care provider orders them to see if you need medical treatment. You pay 20% of the Medicare-approved amount, and the Part B deductible applies. In a hospital outpatient setting, you also pay the hospital a copayment.

Note: Original Medicare doesn't cover hearing aids or exams for fitting hearing aids.

Hepatitis B Shots

Medicare covers these shots for people at high or medium risk for Hepatitis B. Your risk for Hepatitis B increases if you have hemophilia, End-Stage Renal Disease (ESRD), or certain conditions that increase your risk for infection. Other factors may increase your risk for Hepatitis B, so check with your doctor or other health care provider. You pay nothing for the shot if the doctor or other health care provider accepts assignment.

HIV Screening

Medicare covers HIV (Human Immunodeficiency Virus) screening for people at increased risk for the infection, anyone who asks for the test, and pregnant women. Medicare covers this test once every 12 months or up to 3 times during a pregnancy. You pay nothing for the HIV screening.

Part B-Covered Services

Home Health Services

Medicare covers medically-necessary part-time or intermittent skilled nursing care, and/or physical therapy, speech-language pathology services, and/or services for people with a continuing need for occupational therapy. A doctor enrolled in Medicare, or certain health care providers who work with the doctor, must see you face-to-face before the doctor can certify that you need home health services. That doctor must order your care, and a Medicare-certified home health agency must provide it.

Home health services may also include medical social services, part-time or intermittent home health aide services, durable medical equipment, and medical supplies for use at home. You must be homebound, which means leaving home is a major effort. You pay nothing for covered home health services. For Medicare-covered durable medical equipment information, see page 42.

Kidney Dialysis Services and Supplies

Generally, Medicare covers dialysis treatment three times a week if you have End-Stage Renal Disease (ESRD). This includes dialysis medications, laboratory tests, home dialysis training, and related equipment and supplies. The dialysis facility is responsible for coordinating your dialysis services (at home or in a facility). You pay 20% of the Medicare-approved amount and the Part B deductible applies.

Kidney Disease Education Services

Medicare may cover up to six sessions of kidney disease education services if you have Stage IV kidney disease, and your doctor or other health care provider refers you for the service. You pay 20% of the Medicare-approved amount, and the Part B deductible applies.

Laboratory Services

Medicare covers laboratory services including certain blood tests, urinalysis, and some screening tests. You pay nothing for these services.

Part B-Covered Services

Medical Nutrition Therapy Services

Medicare may cover medical nutrition therapy and certain related services if you have diabetes or kidney disease, or you have had a kidney transplant in the last 36 months, and your doctor or other health care provider refers you for the service. You pay nothing for these services if the doctor or other health care provider accepts assignment.

Mental Health Care (outpatient)

Medicare covers mental health care services to help with conditions such as depression or anxiety. Coverage includes services generally provided in an outpatient setting (such as a doctor's or other health care provider's office or hospital outpatient department), including visits with a psychiatrist or other doctor, clinical psychologist, nurse practitioner, physician's assistant, clinical nurse specialist, or clinical social worker; certain treatment for substance abuse; and lab tests. Certain limits and conditions apply.

What you pay will depend on whether you're being diagnosed and monitored or whether you're getting treatment.

- For visits to a doctor or other health care provider to diagnose your condition, you pay 20% of the Medicare-approved amount.
- Generally, for outpatient treatment of your condition (such as counseling or psychotherapy), you pay 40% of the Medicare-approved amount. This coinsurance amount will decrease until it reaches 20% in 2014.

The Part B deductible applies for both visits to diagnose or treat your condition.

Note: Inpatient mental health care is covered under Part A. See Hospital Care (Inpatient) on page 34.

Talk to your doctor or other health care provider if you feel sad, have little interest in things you used to enjoy, feel dependent on drugs or alcohol, or have thoughts about ending your life.

Occupational Therapy

Medicare covers evaluation and treatment to help you perform activities of daily living (such as dressing or bathing) after an illness or accident when your doctor or other health care provider certifies you need it. There may be a limit on the amount Medicare will pay for these services in a single year and there may be certain exceptions to these limits. You pay 20% of the Medicare-approved amount, and the Part B deductible applies.

Part B-Covered Services

Outpatient Hospital Services

Medicare covers many diagnostic and treatment services in participating hospital outpatient departments. Generally, you pay 20% of the Medicare-approved amount for the doctor's or other health care provider's services. You may pay more for services you get in a hospital outpatient setting than you will pay for the same care in a doctor's office. In addition to the amount you pay the doctor, you will usually pay the hospital a copayment for each service you get in a hospital outpatient setting, except for certain preventive services for which there is no copayment. The copayment can't be more than the Part A hospital stay deductible. The Part B deductible applies.

Outpatient Medical and Surgical Services and Supplies

Medicare covers approved procedures like X-rays, casts, or stitches. You pay 20% of the Medicare-approved amount for the doctor's or other health care provider's services. You generally pay the hospital a copayment for each service you get in a hospital outpatient setting. For each service, the copayment can't be more than the Part A hospital stay deductible. The Part B deductible applies, and you pay all charges for items or services that Medicare doesn't cover.

Physical Therapy

Medicare covers evaluation and treatment for injuries and diseases that change your ability to function when your doctor or other health care provider certifies your need for it. There may be a limit on the amount Medicare will pay for these services in a single year and there may be certain exceptions to these limits. You pay 20% of the Medicare-approved amount, and the Part B deductible applies.

Pneumococcal Shot

Medicare covers pneumococcal shots to help prevent pneumococcal infections (like certain types of pneumonia). Most people only need this shot once in their lifetime. Talk with your doctor or other health care provider to see if you should get this shot. You pay nothing if the doctor or other health care provider accepts assignment for giving the shot.

Part B-Covered Services

Prescription Drugs (limited)

Medicare covers a limited number of drugs such as injections you get in a doctor's office, certain oral cancer drugs, drugs used with some types of durable medical equipment (like a nebulizer or external infusion pump), and under very limited circumstances, certain drugs you get in a hospital outpatient setting. You pay 20% of the Medicare-approved amount for these covered drugs.

If the covered drugs you get in a hospital outpatient setting are part of your outpatient services, you pay the copayment for the services. However, other types of drugs in a hospital outpatient setting (sometimes called "self-administered drugs" or drugs you would normally take on your own), aren't covered by Part B. What you pay depends on whether you have Part D or other prescription drug coverage, whether your drug plan covers the drug, and whether the hospital's pharmacy is in your drug plan's network. Contact your prescription drug plan to find out what you pay for drugs you get in a hospital outpatient setting that aren't covered under Part B. See page 94 for more information.

Other than the examples above, you pay 100% for most prescription drugs, unless you have Part D or other drug coverage.

Prostate Cancer Screenings

Medicare covers a Prostate Specific Antigen (PSA) test and a digital rectal exam once every 12 months for men over 50 (beginning the day after your 50th birthday). You pay nothing for the PSA test. You pay 20% of the Medicare-approved amount, and the Part B deductible applies for the digital rectal exam. In a hospital outpatient setting, you also pay the hospital a copayment.

Prosthetic/Orthotic Items

Medicare covers arm, leg, back, and neck braces; artificial eyes; artificial limbs (and their replacement parts); some types of breast prostheses (after mastectomy); and prosthetic devices needed to replace an internal body part or function (including ostomy supplies, and parenteral and enteral nutrition therapy) when ordered by a doctor or other health care provider enrolled in Medicare. For Medicare to cover your prosthetic or orthotic, you must go to a supplier that's enrolled in Medicare. You pay 20% of the Medicare-approved amount, and the Part B deductible applies.

Part B-Covered Services

Pulmonary Rehabilitation

Medicare covers a comprehensive pulmonary rehabilitation program if you have moderate to very severe chronic obstructive pulmonary disease (COPD) and have a referral from the doctor treating this chronic respiratory disease. You pay 20% of the Medicare-approved amount if you get the service in a doctor's office. You also pay the hospital a copayment per session if you get the service in a hospital outpatient setting. The Part B deductible applies.

Rural Health Clinic Services

Medicare covers many outpatient primary care and preventive services in rural health clinics. Generally, you pay 20% of the Medicare-approved amount and the Part B deductible applies. However, you pay nothing for most preventive services.

Second Surgical Opinions

Medicare covers second surgical opinions in some cases for surgery that isn't an emergency. In some cases, Medicare covers third surgical opinions. You pay 20% of the Medicare-approved amount, and the Part B deductible applies.

Speech-Language Pathology Services

Medicare covers evaluation and treatment given to regain and strengthen speech and language skills, including cognitive and swallowing skills, when your doctor or other health care provider certifies you need it. There may be a limit on the amount Medicare will pay for these services in a single year, and there may be certain exceptions to these limits. You pay 20% of the Medicare-approved amount, and the Part B deductible applies.

Surgical Dressing Services

Medicare covers these services for treatment of a surgical or surgically-treated wound. You pay 20% of the Medicare-approved amount for the doctor's or other health care provider's services. You pay a fixed copayment for these services when you get them in a hospital outpatient setting. You pay nothing for the supplies. The Part B deductible applies.

Part B-Covered Services

Tobacco Use Cessation Counseling

If you're diagnosed with an illness caused or complicated by tobacco use, or you take a medicine that's affected by tobacco, Medicare covers up to 8 face-to-face visits in a 12-month period. You pay 20% of the Medicare-approved amount, and the Part B deductible applies. In a hospital outpatient setting, you also pay the hospital a copayment.

If you haven't been diagnosed with an illness caused or complicated by tobacco use, Medicare coverage of tobacco use cessation counseling is considered a covered preventive service. You pay nothing for the counseling sessions if the doctor or other health care provider accepts assignment.

Telehealth

Medicare covers limited medical or other health services, like office visits and consultations provided using an interactive two-way telecommunications system (like real-time audio and video) by an eligible provider who isn't at your location. These services are available in some rural areas, under certain conditions, and only if you're located at one of the following places: a doctor's office, hospital, rural health clinic, federally-qualified health center, hospital-based dialysis facility, skilled nursing facility, or community mental health center. For most of these services, you pay 20% of the Medicare-approved amount, and the Part B deductible applies.

Tests (other than lab tests)

Medicare covers X-rays, MRIs, CT scans, EKGs, and some other diagnostic tests. You pay 20% of the Medicare-approved amount, and the Part B deductible applies. If you get the test at a hospital as an outpatient, you also pay the hospital a copayment that may be more than 20% of the Medicare-approved amount, but it can't be more than the Part A hospital stay deductible. See Laboratory Services on page 45 for other Part B-covered tests.

Part B-Covered Services

Transplants and Immunosuppressive Drugs

Medicare covers doctor services for heart, lung, kidney, pancreas, intestine, and liver transplants under certain conditions and only in a Medicare-certified facility. Medicare covers bone marrow and cornea transplants under certain conditions.

Medicare covers immunosuppressive drugs if the transplant was eligible for Medicare payment, or an employer or union group health plan was required to pay before Medicare paid for the transplant. You must have Part A at the time of the transplant, and you must have Part B at the time you get immunosuppressive drugs. You pay 20% of the Medicare-approved amount, and the Part B deductible applies.

If you're thinking about joining a Medicare Advantage Plan (like an HMO or PPO) and are on a transplant waiting list or believe you need a transplant, check with the plan before you join to make sure your doctors, other health care providers, and hospitals are in the plan's network. Also, check the plan's coverage rules for prior authorization.

Note: Medicare drug plans (Part D) may cover immunosuppressive drugs, even if Medicare or an employer or union group health plan didn't pay for the transplant.

Part B-Covered Services

Travel (health care needed when traveling outside the United States)

Medicare generally doesn't cover health care while you're traveling outside the U.S. (the "U.S." includes the 50 states, the District of Columbia, Puerto Rico, the U.S. Virgin Islands, Guam, the Northern Mariana Islands, and American Samoa). There are some exceptions including some cases where Medicare may pay for services that you get while on board a ship within the territorial waters adjoining the land areas of the U.S. Medicare may pay for inpatient hospital, doctor, or ambulance services you get in a foreign country in the following rare cases:

1. You're in the U.S. when an emergency occurs and the foreign hospital is closer than the nearest U.S. hospital that can treat your medical condition.
2. You're traveling through Canada without unreasonable delay by the most direct route between Alaska and another state when a medical emergency occurs and the Canadian hospital is closer than the nearest U.S. hospital that can treat the emergency.
3. You live in the U.S. and the foreign hospital is closer to your home than the nearest U.S. hospital that can treat your medical condition, regardless of whether an emergency exists.

Medicare may cover medically-necessary ambulance transportation to a foreign hospital only with admission for medically-necessary covered inpatient hospital services.

You pay 20% of the Medicare-approved amount, and the Part B deductible applies.

Urgently-Needed Care

Medicare covers urgently-needed care to treat a sudden illness or injury that isn't a medical emergency. You pay 20% of the Medicare-approved amount for the doctor's or other health care provider's services and the Part B deductible applies. In a hospital outpatient setting, you also pay the hospital a copayment.

Blue words in the text are defined on pages 141–144.

Part B-Covered Services

"Welcome to Medicare" Preventive Visit

During the first 12 months that you have Part B, you can get a "Welcome to Medicare" preventive visit. This visit helps you and your doctor or other health care provider develop a personalized plan to prevent disease, improve your health, and help you stay well. When you make your appointment, let your doctor's office know that you would like to schedule your "Welcome to Medicare" preventive visit.

Yearly "Wellness" Visit

If you've had Part B for longer than 12 months, you can get a yearly "Wellness" visit to develop or update a personalized plan to prevent disease based on your current health and risk factors. This visit is covered once every 12 months.

Your provider may suggest that you fill out a short questionnaire, called a Health Risk Assessment, as part of this visit. Answering these questions can help you figure out what to work on to stay healthy. The questions are based on years of medical research and advice from the Centers for Disease Control and Prevention (CDC). For more information about the Health Risk Assessment, visit www.medicare.gov.

Note: Your first yearly "Wellness" visit can't take place within 12 months of you having Medicare or your "Welcome to Medicare" visit. However, you don't need to have a "Welcome to Medicare" visit before your yearly "Wellness" visit.

You pay nothing for the "Welcome to Medicare" preventive visit or the yearly "Wellness" visit if the doctor or other health care provider accepts assignment. However if your doctor or other health care provider performs additional tests or services during the same visit that aren't covered under these preventive benefits, you may have to pay coinsurance, and the Part B deductible may apply.

What's NOT Covered by Part A and Part B?

Medicare doesn't cover everything. If you need certain services that Medicare doesn't cover, you will have to pay for them yourself unless one of the following applies to you:

- You have other insurance (including Medicaid) to cover the costs.
- You're in a Medicare health plan that covers these services.

Even if Medicare covers a service or item, you generally have to pay deductibles, coinsurance, and copayments.

Some of the items and services that Medicare doesn't cover include the following:

- Long-term care (also called custodial care). See pages 122–124.
- Routine dental care.
- Dentures.
- Cosmetic surgery.
- Acupuncture.
- Hearing aids.
- Exams for fitting hearing aids.

If you have Original Medicare, to find out if Medicare covers a service you need, visit www.medicare.gov/coverage or call 1-800-MEDICARE (1-800-633-4227). TTY users should call 1-877-486-2048. If you're in a Medicare health plan, contact your plan.

Your Medicare Choices

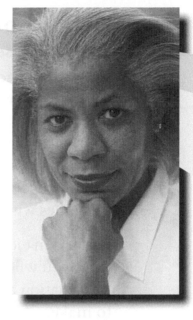

Section 3 includes information about the following:

This handbook has basic information. You will need more detailed information than this handbook provides to make an informed choice. Before making any decisions, learn as much as you can about the types of coverage available to you. See page 56 to get help with your Medicare decisions.

Decide How to Get Your Medicare

You can choose different ways to get your Medicare coverage.

1. You can choose Original Medicare and if you want prescription drug coverage, you must also join a Medicare Prescription Drug Plan (Part D).

2. You can choose to join a Medicare Advantage Plan (like an HMO or PPO), and the plan may include Medicare prescription drug coverage. In most cases, you must take the drug coverage that comes with the Medicare Advantage Plan.

If you don't join a Medicare Advantage Plan or other Medicare health plan, you will have Original Medicare. See the next page for more information about your coverage choices, and the decisions you need to make.

Note: If you have End-Stage Renal Disease (ESRD), you will usually get your health care through Original Medicare. See page 59.

Each year in the fall, you should review your health and prescription needs because your health, finances, or plan's coverage may have changed. If you decide other coverage will better meet your needs, **you can switch plans between October 15–December 7**. See pages 78 and 85. If you're satisfied with your current plan's coverage for the following year, you don't need to do anything.

Need Help Deciding?

1. Visit the Medicare Plan Finder at www.medicare.gov/find-a-plan to find and compare plans in your area.

2. Get free personalized counseling about choosing coverage. See pages 137–140 for the phone number of your State Health Insurance Assistance Program (SHIP).

3. Call 1-800-MEDICARE (1-800-633-4227), and say "Agent." TTY users should call 1-877-486-2048. If you need help in a language other than English or Spanish, let the customer service representative know.

See pages 114–115 to find out how Original Medicare or a Medicare plan you may join uses and releases your personal information.

Blue words in the text are defined on pages 141–144.

Your Medicare Coverage Choices

There are two main choices for how you get your Medicare coverage. Use these steps to help you decide.

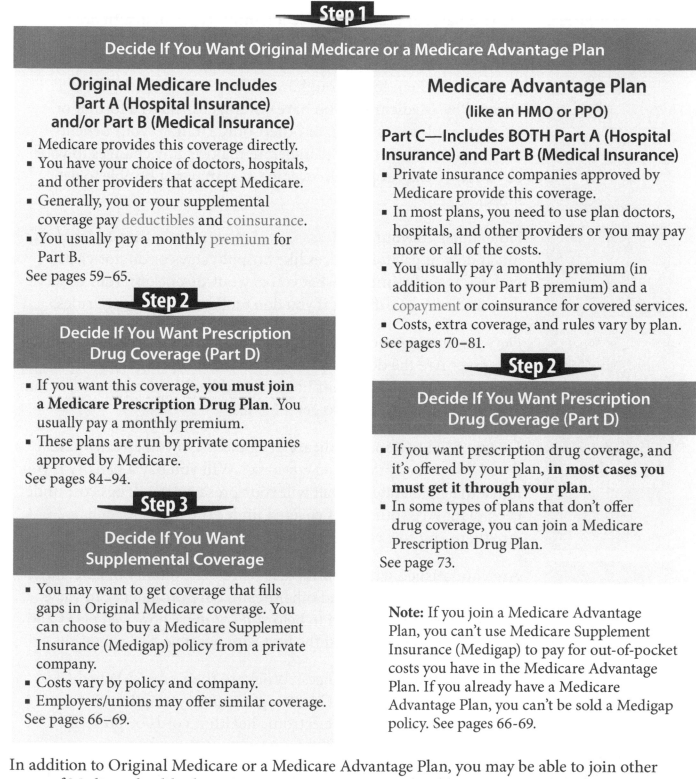

Step 1

Decide If You Want Original Medicare or a Medicare Advantage Plan

Original Medicare Includes
Part A (Hospital Insurance)
and/or Part B (Medical Insurance)

- Medicare provides this coverage directly.
- You have your choice of doctors, hospitals, and other providers that accept Medicare.
- Generally, you or your supplemental coverage pay deductibles and coinsurance.
- You usually pay a monthly premium for Part B.

See pages 59–65.

Medicare Advantage Plan
(like an HMO or PPO)

Part C—Includes BOTH Part A (Hospital Insurance) and Part B (Medical Insurance)

- Private insurance companies approved by Medicare provide this coverage.
- In most plans, you need to use plan doctors, hospitals, and other providers or you may pay more or all of the costs.
- You usually pay a monthly premium (in addition to your Part B premium) and a copayment or coinsurance for covered services.
- Costs, extra coverage, and rules vary by plan.

See pages 70–81.

Step 2

Decide If You Want Prescription Drug Coverage (Part D)

- If you want this coverage, **you must join a Medicare Prescription Drug Plan.** You usually pay a monthly premium.
- These plans are run by private companies approved by Medicare.

See pages 84–94.

Step 2

Decide If You Want Prescription Drug Coverage (Part D)

- If you want prescription drug coverage, and it's offered by your plan, **in most cases you must get it through your plan.**
- In some types of plans that don't offer drug coverage, you can join a Medicare Prescription Drug Plan.

See page 73.

Step 3

Decide If You Want Supplemental Coverage

- You may want to get coverage that fills gaps in Original Medicare coverage. You can choose to buy a Medicare Supplement Insurance (Medigap) policy from a private company.
- Costs vary by policy and company.
- Employers/unions may offer similar coverage.

See pages 66–69.

Note: If you join a Medicare Advantage Plan, you can't use Medicare Supplement Insurance (Medigap) to pay for out-of-pocket costs you have in the Medicare Advantage Plan. If you already have a Medicare Advantage Plan, you can't be sold a Medigap policy. See pages 66-69.

In addition to Original Medicare or a Medicare Advantage Plan, you may be able to join other types of Medicare health plans. See pages 82–83. You may be able to save money or have other choices if you have limited income and resources. See pages 98–104. You may also have other coverage, like employer or union, military, or Veterans' benefits. See pages 95–96.

Things to Consider When Choosing or Changing Your Coverage

Coverage	Are the services you need covered?
Your other coverage	Do you have, or are you eligible for, other types of health or prescription drug coverage (like from a former or current employer or union)? If so, read the materials from your insurer or plan, or call them to find out how the coverage works with, or is affected by, Medicare. If you have coverage through a former or current employer or union or other source, talk to your benefits administrator, insurer, or plan before making any changes to your coverage. If you drop your coverage, you may not be able to get it back.
Cost	How much are your premiums, deductibles, and other costs? How much do you pay for services like hospital stays or doctor visits? Is there a yearly limit on what you pay out-of-pocket? Your costs vary and may be different if you don't follow the coverage rules.
Doctor and hospital choice	Do your doctors and other health care providers accept the coverage? Are the doctors you want to see accepting new patients? Do you have to choose your hospital and health care providers from a network? Do you need to get referrals?
Prescription drugs	Do you need to join a Medicare drug plan? Do you already have creditable prescription drug coverage? Will you pay a penalty if you join a drug plan later? What will your prescription drugs cost under each plan? Are your drugs covered under the plan's formulary? Are there any coverage rules that apply to your prescriptions?
Quality of care	Are you satisfied with your medical care? The quality of care and services given by plans and other health care providers can vary. Medicare has information to help you compare how well plans and providers work to give you the best care possible. See page 131.
Convenience	Where are the doctors' offices? What are their hours? Which pharmacies can you use? Can you get your prescriptions by mail? Do the doctors use electronic health records or prescribe electronically? See page 132.
Travel	Will the plan cover you in another state or outside the U.S.?

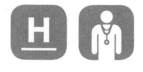

Original Medicare

Original Medicare is one of your health coverage choices as part of the Medicare Program. You will be in Original Medicare unless you choose a Medicare health plan.

How Does It Work?

Original Medicare is coverage managed by the Federal government. Generally, there is a cost for each service. Here are the general rules for how it works:

	Original Medicare
Can I get my health care from any doctor, other health care provider, or hospital?	In most cases, yes. You can go to any doctor, other health care provider, hospital, or other facility that's enrolled in Medicare and is accepting new Medicare patients.
Are prescription drugs covered?	With a few exceptions (see pages 34 and 48), most prescriptions aren't covered. You can add drug coverage by joining a Medicare Prescription Drug Plan (Part D).
Do I need to choose a primary care doctor?	No.
Do I have to get a referral to see a specialist?	In most cases no, but the specialist must be enrolled in Medicare.
Should I get a supplemental policy?	You may already have employer or union coverage that may pay costs that Original Medicare doesn't. If not, you may want to buy a Medicare Supplement Insurance (Medigap) policy. See pages 66–69.
What else do I need to know about Original Medicare?	■ You generally pay a set amount for your health care (deductible) before Medicare pays its share. Then, Medicare pays its share, and you pay your share (coinsurance/copayment) for covered services and supplies. There is no yearly limit for what you pay out-of-pocket. ■ You usually pay a monthly premium for Part B. See page 102 for more information about Medicare Savings Programs for help paying your Part B premium. ■ You generally don't need to file Medicare claims. The law requires providers (like doctors, hospitals, skilled nursing facilities, and home health agencies) and suppliers to file your claims for the covered services and supplies you get.

Blue words in the text are defined on pages 141–144.

What You Pay

Your out-of-pocket costs in Original Medicare depend on the following:

- Whether you have Part A and/or Part B. Most people have both.
- Whether your doctor, other health care provider, or supplier accepts "assignment."
- The type of health care you need and how often you need it.
- Whether you choose to get services or supplies Medicare doesn't cover. If you do, you pay all the costs unless you have other insurance that covers it.
- Whether you have other health insurance that works with Medicare.
- Whether you have Medicaid or get state help paying your Medicare costs. See pages 102–103.
- Whether you have a Medicare Supplement Insurance (Medigap) policy.
- Whether you and your doctor or other health care provider sign a private contract. See page 64.

For more information on how other insurance works with Medicare, see pages 26–27. For more information about help to cover the costs that Original Medicare doesn't cover, see page 97.

Medicare Summary Notices

If you get a Medicare-covered service, you will get a Medicare Summary Notice (MSN) in the mail every 3 months. The notice shows all your services or supplies that providers and suppliers billed to Medicare during the 3-month period, what Medicare paid, and what you may owe the provider. **This notice isn't a bill.** Read it carefully and do the following:

- If you have other insurance, check to see if it covers anything that Medicare didn't.

- Keep your receipts and bills, and compare them to your notice to be sure you got all the services, supplies, or equipment listed. See pages 117–119 for information on Medicare fraud.

- If you paid a bill before you got your notice, compare your notice with the bill to make sure you paid the right amount for your services.

- If an item or service is denied, call your doctor's or other health care provider's office to make sure they submitted the correct information. If not, the office may resubmit.

If you disagree with any decision made, you can file an appeal, see pages 107–108.

If you need to change your address on your notice, call Social Security at 1-800-772-1213. TTY users should call 1-800-325-0778. If you get Railroad Retirement Board (RRB) benefits, call the RRB at 1-877-772-5772.

You don't have to wait for your MSN to view your Medicare claims. Visit www.MyMedicare.gov to look at your Medicare claims or view electronic MSNs. See page 130. Your claims generally will be available for viewing within 24 hours after processing.

Keeping Your Costs Down with "Assignment"

Assignment means that your doctor, provider, or supplier agrees (or is required by law) to accept the Medicare-approved amount as full payment for covered services. Some health care providers who are enrolled in Medicare have signed an agreement to accept assignment for all Medicare-covered services. They are called "participating" providers. Other health care providers haven't signed an agreement to accept assignment for all Medicare-covered services, but they can still choose to accept assignment for individual services. These providers are called "non-participating."

Most doctors, providers, and suppliers accept assignment, but you should always check to make sure. Find out how much you have to pay for each service or supply before you get it.

Here's what happens if your doctor, provider, or supplier **accepts** assignment:

- Your out-of-pocket costs may be less.
- They agree to charge you only the Medicare deductible and coinsurance amount and usually wait for Medicare to pay its share before asking you to pay your share.
- They have to submit your claim directly to Medicare and can't charge you for submitting the claim.

Blue words in the text are defined on pages 141–144.

Keeping Your Costs Down with "Assignment" (continued)

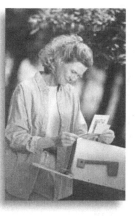

Here's what happens if your doctor, provider, or supplier **doesn't accept** assignment:

- You might have to pay the entire charge at the time of service. Your doctor, provider, or supplier is supposed to submit a claim to Medicare for any Medicare-covered services they provide to you. They can't charge you for submitting a claim. If they don't submit the Medicare claim once you ask them to, call 1-800-MEDICARE (1-800-633-4227). TTY users should call 1-877-486-2048.

  Note: In some cases, you might have to submit your own claim to Medicare using form CMS-1490S to get paid back. Visit www.medicare.gov/medicareonlineforms for the form and instructions or call 1-800-MEDICARE.

- They can charge you more than the Medicare-approved amount, but there is a limit called "the limiting charge." The provider can only charge you up to 15% over the amount that non-participating providers are paid. Non-participating providers are paid 95% of the fee schedule amount. The limiting charge applies only to certain Medicare-covered services and doesn't apply to some supplies and durable medical equipment.

To find out if your doctors and other health care providers accept assignment or participate in Medicare, visit www.medicare.gov/physician or www.medicare.gov/supplier. You can also call 1-800-MEDICARE, or ask your doctor, provider, or supplier if they accept assignment.

What to Know About Private Contracts

A "private contract" is a written agreement between you and a doctor or other health care provider who has decided not to provide services to anyone through Medicare. The private contract only applies to the services provided by the doctor or other provider who asked you to sign it. You don't have to sign a private contract. You can always go to another provider who gives services through Medicare. If you sign a private contract with your doctor or other provider, the following rules apply:

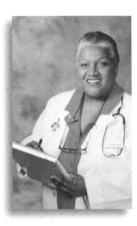

- **Medicare won't pay any amount for the services you get from this doctor or provider, even if it's a Medicare-covered service.**
- You will have to pay the full amount of whatever this provider charges you for the services you get.
- If you have a Medicare Supplement Insurance (Medigap) policy, it won't pay anything for the services you get. Call your insurance company before you get the service if you have questions.
- Your provider must tell you if Medicare would pay for the service if you got it from another provider who accepts Medicare.
- Your provider must tell you if he or she has been excluded from Medicare.

You can't be asked to sign a private contract for emergency or urgent care.

You're always free to get services not covered by Medicare if you choose to pay for a service yourself.

You may want to contact your State Health Insurance Assistance Program (SHIP) to get help before signing a private contract with any doctor or other health care provider. See pages 137–140 for the phone number.

 See pages 107–119 for information about your appeal rights and how to protect yourself and Medicare from fraud.

Adding Medicare Drug Coverage (Part D)

In Original Medicare, **if you don't already have** creditable prescription drug coverage (for example, from a current or former employer or union) and you would like Medicare prescription drug coverage, you must join a Medicare Prescription Drug Plan. These plans are available through private companies under contract with Medicare. If you don't currently have creditable prescription drug coverage, you should think about joining a Medicare Prescription Drug Plan as soon as you're eligible. **If you don't join a Medicare Prescription Drug Plan when you're first eligible and you decide to join later, you may have to pay a late enrollment penalty.** See pages 90–91 for more information.

If you have creditable prescription drug coverage from an employer or union, call your employer or union's benefits administrator before you make any changes to your coverage. Your employer or union plan will tell you each year if your prescription drug coverage is creditable prescription drug coverage. If you drop your employer or union coverage, you may not be able to get it back. You also may not be able to drop your employer or union **drug** coverage without also dropping your employer or union **health** (doctor and hospital) coverage. If you drop coverage for yourself, you may also have to drop coverage for your spouse and dependants.

Extra Help Paying for Coverage

People with limited income and resources may qualify for Extra Help paying their Medicare prescription drug coverage costs. See pages 98–101 to find out if you may qualify for Extra Help.

Blue words in the text are defined on pages 141–144.

Medicare Supplement Insurance (Medigap) Policies

Original Medicare pays for many, but not all, health care services and supplies. A Medicare Supplement Insurance policy, sold by private companies, can help pay some of the health care costs that Original Medicare doesn't cover, like copayments, coinsurance, and deductibles. **Medicare Supplement Insurance policies are also called Medigap policies.**

Some Medigap policies also offer coverage for services that Original Medicare doesn't cover, like medical care when you travel outside the U.S. If you have Original Medicare and you buy a Medigap policy, Medicare will pay its share of the Medicare-approved amount for covered health care costs. Then your Medigap policy pays its share. You have to pay the premiums for a Medigap policy.

Every Medigap policy must follow Federal and state laws designed to protect you, and it must be clearly identified as "Medicare Supplement Insurance." Insurance companies can sell you only a "standardized" policy identified in most states by letters A–N. All policies offer the same basic benefits but some offer additional benefits, so you can choose which one meets your needs. In Massachusetts, Minnesota, and Wisconsin, Medigap policies are standardized in a different way.

Note: Plans E, H, I, and J are no longer available to buy, but if you already have one of those policies, you can keep it. Contact your insurance company for more information.

Different insurance companies may charge different premiums for the same exact policy. As you shop for a policy, be sure you're comparing the same policy (for example, compare Plan A from one company with Plan A from another company).

In some states, you may be able to buy another type of Medigap policy called Medicare SELECT (a policy that requires you to use specific hospitals and, in some cases, specific doctors or other health care providers to get full coverage). If you buy a Medigap SELECT policy, you have the right to change your mind within 12 months and switch to a standard Medigap policy.

Blue words in the text are defined on pages 141–144.

The chart below shows basic information about the different benefits that Medigap policies cover. If a check mark appears, the plan covers the described benefit 100%. If a percentage appears, the plan covers that percentage of the benefit.

Note: You will need more details than this chart provides to compare and choose a policy. For more details, visit www.medicare.gov/publications to view the booklet "Choosing a Medigap Policy: A Guide to Health Insurance for People with Medicare." You can also call 1-800-MEDICARE (1-800-633-4227) to find out if a copy can be mailed to you. TTY users should call 1-877-486-2048.

Benefits	Medicare Supplement Insurance Plans (Medigap)									
	A	B	C	D	F*	G	K	L	M	N
Medicare Part A Coinsurance and Hospital Costs (up to an additional 365 days after Medicare benefits are used)	√	√	√	√	√	√	√	√	√	√
Medicare Part B Coinsurance or Copayment	√	√	√	√	√	√	50%	75%	√	√**
Blood (first 3 pints)	√	√	√	√	√	√	50%	75%		
Part A Hospice Care Coinsurance or Copayment	√	√	√	√	√	√	50%	75%	√	√
Skilled Nursing Facility Care Coinsurance			√	√	√	√	50%	75%	√	√
Medicare Part A Deductible		√	√	√	√	√	50%	75%	50%	√
Medicare Part B Deductible			√		√					
Medicare Part B Excess Charges					√	√				
Foreign Travel Emergency (up to plan limits)			√	√	√	√			√	√
							Out-of-Pocket Limit			
							$4,640	$2,320		

* Plan F also offers a high-deductible plan. If you choose this option, this means you must pay for Medicare-covered costs (coinsurance, copayments, deductibles) up to the deductible amount of $2,000 in 2011 before your policy pays anything.

** Plan N pays 100% of the Part B coinsurance, except for a copayment of up to $20 for some office visits and up to a $50 copayment for emergency room visits that don't result in an inpatient admission.

More About Medicare Supplement Insurance (Medigap)

Important Facts

- You must have Part A and Part B.

- You pay a monthly premium for your Medigap policy in addition to your monthly Part B premium.

- A Medigap policy only covers one person. Spouses must buy separate policies.

- You can't have prescription drug coverage in both your Medigap policy and a Medicare drug plan. See page 95.

- It's important to compare Medigap policies since the costs can vary and may go up as you get older. Some states limit Medigap costs.

When to Buy

- The best time to buy a Medigap policy is during the 6-month period that begins on the first day of the month in which you're 65 or older **and** enrolled in Part B. (Some states have additional open enrollment periods.) After this enrollment period, your option to buy a Medigap policy may be limited and it may cost more. For example, if you turn 65 and are enrolled in Part B in June, the best time for you to buy a Medigap policy is from June to November.

- If you have group health coverage based on your (or your spouse's) current employment, your Medigap Open Enrollment Period will start when you sign up for Part B.

- Federal law doesn't require insurance companies to sell Medigap policies to people under 65. If you're under 65, you might not be able to buy the Medigap policy you want, or any Medigap policy, until you turn 65. However, some states require Medigap insurance companies to sell you a Medigap policy, even if you're under 65.

If You're in a Medicare Advantage Plan

- If you have a Medigap policy and join a Medicare Advantage Plan (like an HMO or PPO), you may want to drop your Medigap policy. Your Medigap policy **can't** be used to pay your Medicare Advantage Plan copayments, deductibles, and premiums. If you want to cancel your Medigap policy, contact your insurance company. In most cases, if you drop your Medigap policy to join a Medicare Advantage Plan, you won't be able to get it back.

Blue words in the text are defined on pages 141–144.

If You're in a Medicare Advantage Plan (continued)

- If you have a Medicare Advantage Plan, it's illegal for anyone to sell you a Medigap policy unless you're switching back to Original Medicare. Contact your State Insurance Department if this happens to you. If you want to switch to Original Medicare and buy a Medigap policy, contact your Medicare Advantage Plan to disenroll.

- If you join a Medicare Advantage Plan for the first time, and you aren't happy with the plan, you will have special rights to buy a Medigap policy if you return to Original Medicare within 12 months of joining.
  - If you had a Medigap policy before you joined, you may be able to get the same policy back if the company still sells it. If it isn't available, you can buy another Medigap policy.
  - The Medigap policy can no longer have prescription drug coverage even if you had it before, but you may be able to join a Medicare Prescription Drug Plan.
  - If you joined a Medicare Advantage Plan when you were first eligible for Medicare, you can choose from any Medigap policy.

For More Information About Medicare Supplement Insurance (Medigap)

- Visit www.medicare.gov/publications to view the booklet "Choosing a Medigap Policy: A Guide to Health Insurance for People with Medicare." You can also call 1-800-MEDICARE (1-800-633-4227) to find out if a copy can be mailed to you. TTY users should call 1-877-486-2048.
- Visit www.medicare.gov/Medigap.
- Call your State Insurance Department. Visit www.medicare.gov/contacts or call 1-800-MEDICARE to get the phone number.
- Call your State Health Insurance Assistance Program (SHIP). See pages 137–140 for the phone number.

Medicare Advantage Plans (Part C)

A Medicare Advantage Plan (like an HMO or PPO) is another Medicare health plan choice you may have as part of Medicare. Medicare Advantage Plans, sometimes called "Part C" or "MA Plans," are offered by private companies approved by Medicare. If you join a Medicare Advantage Plan, you still have Medicare. You will get your Part A (Hospital Insurance) and Part B (Medical Insurance) coverage from the Medicare Advantage Plan and not Original Medicare. In all types of Medicare Advantage Plans, you're always covered for emergency and urgent care. Medicare Advantage Plans must cover all of the services that Original Medicare covers except hospice care. Original Medicare covers hospice care even if you're in a Medicare Advantage Plan. Medicare Advantage Plans aren't supplemental coverage.

Medicare Advantage Plans may offer extra coverage, such as vision, hearing, dental, and/or health and wellness programs. Most include Medicare prescription drug coverage (Part D). In addition to your Part B premium, you usually pay a monthly premium for the Medicare Advantage Plan.

Medicare pays a fixed amount for your care every month to the companies offering Medicare Advantage Plans. These companies must follow rules set by Medicare. However, each Medicare Advantage Plan can charge different out-of-pocket costs and have different rules for how you get services (like whether you need a referral to see a specialist or if you have to go to only doctors, facilities, or suppliers that belong to the plan for non-emergency or non-urgent care). These rules can change each year.

There are different types of Medicare Advantage Plans:

- Health Maintenance Organization (HMO) Plans—In most HMOs, you can only go to doctors, other health care providers, or hospitals on the plan's list except in an emergency. You may also need to get a referral from your primary care doctor. See page 76.
- Preferred Provider Organization (PPO) Plans—In a PPO, you pay less if you use doctors, hospitals, and other health care providers that belong to the plan's network. You pay more if you use doctors, hospitals, and providers outside of the network. See page 76.

Blue words in the text are defined on pages 141–144.

Medicare Advantage Plans (continued)

- Private Fee-for-Service (PFFS) Plans—PFFS plans are similar to Original Medicare in that you can generally go to any doctor, other health care provider, or hospital as long as they agree to treat you. The plan determines how much it will pay doctors, other health care providers, and hospitals, and how much you must pay when you get care. See page 77.
- Special Needs Plans (SNP)—SNPs provide focused and specialized health care for specific groups of people, such as those who have both Medicare and Medicaid, who live in a nursing home, or have certain chronic medical conditions. See page 77.

There are other less common types of Medicare Advantage Plans that may be available:

- HMO Point-of-Service (HMOPOS) Plans—This is an HMO plan that may allow you to get some services out-of-network for a higher copayment or coinsurance.
- Medical Savings Account (MSA) Plans—This is a plan that combines a high deductible health plan with a bank account. Medicare deposits money into the account (usually less than the deductible). You can use the money to pay for your health care services during the year. For more information about MSAs, visit www.medicare.gov/publications to view the booklet "Your Guide to Medicare Medical Savings Account Plans." You can also call 1-800-MEDICARE (1-800-633-4227) to find out if a copy can be mailed to you. TTY users should call 1-877-486-2048.

Make sure you understand how a plan works before you join. See pages 76–77 for more information about Medicare Advantage Plan types. If you want more information about a Medicare Advantage Plan, you can call any plan and request a Summary of Benefits (SB) document. Contact your State Health Insurance Assistance Program (SHIP) for help comparing plans. See pages 137–140 for the phone number.

More About Medicare Advantage Plans

Important Facts

- As with Original Medicare, you still have Medicare rights and protections, including the right to appeal. See pages 107–109.
- You can check with the plan before you get a service to find out if it's covered and what your costs may be.
- You must follow plan rules, like getting a referral to see a specialist to avoid higher costs if your plan requires it. The specialist you're referred to must also be in the plan's network. Check with the plan.
- If you go to a doctor, other health care provider, facility, or supplier that doesn't belong to the plan, your services may not be covered, or your costs could be higher. In most cases, this applies to Medicare Advantage HMOs and PPOs.
- If you join a clinical research study, some costs may be covered by your plan. Call your plan for more information.
- Medicare Advantage Plans can't charge more than Original Medicare for certain services, like chemotherapy, dialysis, and skilled nursing facility care.
- Medicare Advantage Plans have a yearly cap on how much you pay for Part A and Part B services during the year. This yearly maximum out-of-pocket amount can be different between Medicare Advantage Plans. You should consider this when you choose a plan.

Blue words in the text are defined on pages 141–144.

Joining and Leaving

- You can join a Medicare Advantage Plan even if you have a pre-existing condition, except for End-Stage Renal Disease (ESRD). See page 74.
- You can only join or leave a plan at certain times during the year. See pages 78–79.
- Each year, Medicare Advantage Plans can choose to leave Medicare or make changes to the services they cover and what you pay. If the plan decides to stop participating in Medicare, you will have to join another Medicare health plan or return to Original Medicare. See pages 106–107.

More About Medicare Advantage Plans (continued)

Prescription Drug Coverage

- You usually get prescription drug coverage (Part D) through the plan. In some types of plans that don't offer drug coverage, you can join a Medicare Prescription Drug Plan. **If you're in a Medicare Advantage Plan that includes prescription drug coverage and you join a Medicare Prescription Drug Plan, you will be disenrolled from your Medicare Advantage Plan and returned to Original Medicare.** You can't have prescription drug coverage through both a Medicare Advantage Plan and a Medicare Prescription Drug Plan.

Who Can Join?

To join a Medicare Advantage Plan you must meet these conditions:

- You have Part A and Part B.
- You live in the plan's service area.
- You don't have End-Stage Renal Disease (ESRD) except as explained on page 74.

Note: In most cases, you can join a Medicare Advantage Plan only at certain times during the year. See pages 78–79.

If You Have Other Coverage

Talk to your employer, union, or other benefits administrator about their rules before you join a Medicare Advantage Plan. In some cases, joining a Medicare Advantage Plan might cause you to lose employer or union coverage. If you lose coverage for yourself, you may also lose coverage for your spouse and dependants. In other cases, if you join a Medicare Advantage Plan, you may still be able to use your employer or union coverage along with the plan you join. **Remember, if you drop your employer or union coverage, you may not be able to get it back.**

If You Have a Medicare Supplement Insurance Policy

You don't need to buy (and can't be sold) a Medicare Supplement Insurance (Medigap) policy while you're in a Medicare Advantage Plan. If you already have a Medigap policy and join a Medicare Advantage Plan, you will probably want to drop your Medigap policy. You can't use it to pay for any expenses (copayments, deductibles, and premiums) you have under a Medicare Advantage Plan. If you drop your Medigap policy, you may not be able to get it back. See pages 66–69.

If You Have End-Stage Renal Disease (ESRD)

If you have End-Stage Renal Disease (ESRD), you can only join a Medicare Advantage Plan in certain situations:

- If you're already in a Medicare Advantage Plan when you develop ESRD, you may be able to stay in your plan or join another plan offered by the same company.
- If you have an employer or union health plan or other health coverage through a company that offers Medicare Advantage Plans, you may be able to join one of their Medicare Advantage Plans.
- If you've had a successful kidney transplant, you may be able to join a Medicare Advantage Plan.
- You may be able to join a Medicare Special Needs Plan (SNP) for people with ESRD if one is available in your area.

Your Rights if Your Plan Stops Participating in Medicare

If you have ESRD and are in a Medicare Advantage Plan, and the plan leaves Medicare or no longer provides coverage in your area, you have a one-time right to join another plan. You don't have to use your one-time right to join a new plan immediately. If you go directly to Original Medicare after your plan leaves or stops providing coverage, you will still have a one-time right to join a Medicare Advantage Plan later.

Have Questions or Complaints about Kidney Dialysis Services?

Call your local ESRD Network. ESRD Networks help people with ESRD get the right care at the right time. The Networks make sure that dialysis services are administered effectively, help improve quality of care for people with ESRD, and provide help to people with ESRD including resolving patient grievances. Call 1-800-MEDICARE (1-800-633-4227) to get the phone number for the ESRD Network in your area. TTY users should call 1-877-486-2048.

For More Information

Visit www.medicare.gov/publications to view the booklet "Medicare Coverage of Kidney Dialysis and Kidney Transplant Services." You can also call 1-800-MEDICARE to see if a copy can be mailed to you.

Note: If you have ESRD and Original Medicare, you may join a Medicare Prescription Drug Plan.

What You Pay

Your out-of-pocket costs in a Medicare Advantage Plan depend on the following:

- Whether the plan charges a monthly premium.
- Whether the plan pays any of your monthly Part B premium.
- Whether the plan has a yearly deductible or any additional deductibles.
- How much you pay for each visit or service (copayments or coinsurance).
- The type of health care services you need and how often you get them.
- Whether you go to a doctor or supplier who accepts assignment (if you're in a Preferred Provider Organization, Private Fee-for-Service Plan, or Medical Savings Account Plan and you go out-of-network). See page 62 for more information about assignment.
- Whether you follow the plan's rules, like using network providers.
- Whether you need extra benefits and if the plan charges for it.
- The plan's yearly limit on your out-of-pocket costs for all medical services.
- Whether you have Medicaid or get help from your state.

To learn more about your costs in specific Medicare Advantage Plans, visit www.medicare.gov/find-a-plan. You can also call 1-800-MEDICARE (1-800-633-4227). TTY users should call 1-877-486-2048.

Blue words in the text are defined on pages 141–144.

If you're in a Medicare plan, review the Evidence of Coverage (EOC) and Annual Notice of Change (ANOC) your plan sends you each fall. The EOC gives you details about what the plan covers, how much you pay, and more. The ANOC includes any changes in coverage, costs, or service area that will be effective in January. If you don't get these important documents, contact your plan.

How Do Medicare Advantage Plans Work?

	Health Maintenance Organization (HMO) Plan	Preferred Provider Organization (PPO) Plan
Can I get my health care from any doctor, other health care provider, or hospital?	No. You generally must get your care and services from doctors, other health care providers, or hospitals in the plan's network (except emergency care, out-of-area urgent care, or out-of-area dialysis). In some plans, you may be able to go out-of-network for certain services, usually for a higher cost. This is called an HMO with a point-of-service (POS) option.	In most cases, yes. PPOs have network doctors, other health care providers, and hospitals, but you can also use out-of-network providers for covered services, usually for a higher cost.
Are prescription drugs covered?	In most cases, yes. Ask the plan. If you want Medicare drug coverage, you must join an HMO Plan that offers prescription drug coverage.	In most cases, yes. Ask the plan. If you want Medicare drug coverage, you must join a PPO Plan that offers prescription drug coverage.
Do I need to choose a primary care doctor?	In most cases, yes.	No.
Do I have to get a referral to see a specialist?	In most cases, yes. Certain services, like yearly screening mammograms, don't require a referral.	In most cases, no.
What else do I need to know about this type of plan?	• If your doctor or other health care provider leaves the plan, your plan will notify you. You can choose another doctor in the plan. • If you get health care outside the plan's network, you may have to pay the full cost. • It's important that you follow the plan's rules, like getting prior approval for a certain service when needed.	• There are two types of PPOs: Regional PPOs and Local PPOs. • If your doctor or other health care provider leaves the plan, your plan will notify you. You can choose another doctor in the plan. • If you get health care outside the plan's network, you may have to pay the full cost.

There may be several private companies that offer different types of Medicare Advantage Plans in your area. Each plan can vary. Read individual plan materials carefully to make sure you understand the plan's rules. You may want to contact the plan to find out if the service you need is covered and how much it costs. Visit the Medicare Plan Finder at www.medicare.gov/find-a-plan to find plans in your area. You can also call 1-800-MEDICARE (1-800-633-4227). TTY users should call 1-877-486-2048.

How Do Medicare Advantage Plans Work? (continued)

Private Fee-for-Service (PFFS) Plan	Special Needs Plan (SNP)
In some cases, yes. **You can go to any Medicare-approved doctor, other health care provider, or hospital that accepts the plan's payment terms and agrees to treat you.** Not all providers will. If you join a PFFS Plan that has a network, you can also see any of the network providers who have agreed to always treat plan members. You can also choose an out-of-network doctor, hospital, or other provider, who accepts the plan's terms, but you may pay more.	You generally must get your care and services from doctors, other health care providers, or hospitals in the plan's network (except emergency care, out-of-area urgent care, or out-of-area dialysis).
Sometimes. If your PFFS Plan doesn't offer drug coverage, you can join a Medicare Prescription Drug Plan (Part D) to get coverage.	Yes. All SNPs must provide Medicare prescription drug coverage (Part D).
No.	Generally, yes.
No.	In most cases, yes. Certain services, like yearly screening mammograms, don't require a referral.
<ul><li>PFFS Plans aren't the same as Original Medicare or Medigap.</li><li>The plan decides how much you must pay for services.</li><li>Some PFFS Plans contract with a network of providers who agree to always treat you even if you've never seen them before.</li><li>Out-of-network doctors, hospitals, and other providers may decide not to treat you even if you've seen them before.</li><li>For each service you get, make sure your doctors, hospitals, and other providers agree to treat you under the plan, and accept the plan's payment terms.</li><li>In an emergency, doctors, hospitals, and other providers must treat you.</li></ul>	<ul><li>A plan must limit membership to the following groups: 1) people who live in certain institutions (like a nursing home) or who require nursing care at home, or 2) people who are eligible for both Medicare and Medicaid, or 3) people who have specific chronic or disabling conditions (like diabetes, ESRD, HIV/AIDS, chronic heart failure, or dementia). Plans may further limit membership. You can join a SNP at any time.</li><li>Plans should coordinate the services and providers you need to help you stay healthy and follow doctor's or other health care provider's orders.</li><li>If you have Medicare and Medicaid, your plan should make sure that all of the plan doctors or other health care providers you use accept Medicaid.</li><li>If you live in an institution, make sure that plan providers serve people where you live.</li></ul>

Join, Switch, or Drop a Medicare Advantage Plan

- **When you first become eligible for Medicare,** you can join during the 7-month period that begins 3 months before the month you turn 65, includes the month you turn 65, and ends 3 months after the month you turn 65.

- **If you get Medicare due to a disability,** you can join during the 7-month period that begins 3 months before your 25th month of disability and ends 3 months after your 25th month of disability.

- **NEW—Between October 15–December 7** anyone can join, switch, or drop a Medicare Advantage Plan. This open enrollment period has changed to give you more time to choose and join a plan. Your coverage will begin on January 1, as long as the plan gets your request by December 7.

Making changes to your coverage after December 7

Between January 1–February 14, if you're in a Medicare Advantage Plan, you can leave your plan and switch to Original Medicare. If you switch to Original Medicare during this period, you will have until February 14 to also join a Medicare Prescription Drug Plan to add drug coverage. Your coverage will begin the first day of the month after the plan gets your enrollment form.

During this period, you **can't** do the following:
- Switch from Original Medicare to a Medicare Advantage Plan.
- Switch from one Medicare Advantage Plan to another.
- Switch from one Medicare Prescription Drug Plan to another.
- Join, switch, or drop a Medicare Medical Savings Account Plan.

Join, Switch, or Drop a Medicare Advantage Plan (continued)

Special Enrollment Periods

In most cases, you must stay enrolled for the calendar year starting the date your coverage begins. However, in certain situations, you may be able to join, switch, or drop a Medicare Advantage Plan during a special enrollment period. Contact your plan if any of these situations apply to you:

- You move out of your plan's service area.
- You have Medicaid.
- You qualify for Extra Help. See pages 98–101.
- You live in an institution (like a nursing home).

NEW: 5-Star Special Enrollment Period

Medicare uses information from member satisfaction surveys, plans, and health care providers to give overall performance star ratings to plans. A plan can get a rating between one to five stars. A 5-star rating is considered excellent. These ratings help you compare plans based on quality and performance.

Starting December 8, 2011, you can switch to a 5-star Medicare Advantage Plan at any time during the year.

- The overall plan star ratings are available at www.medicare.gov/find-a-plan.
- You can only join a 5-star Medicare Advantage Plan if one is available in your area.
- You can only use this special enrollment period to switch to a 5-star plan one time each year.
- You can't use this period to join a Medicare Cost Plan. See page 82.

Visit the Medicare Plan Finder at www.medicare.gov/find-a-plan to search for plans. For more information about overall plan ratings, visit www.medicare.gov/publications to view the fact sheet "Use Medicare's Information on Quality to Help You Compare Plans." You can also call 1-800-MEDICARE (1-800-633-4227). TTY users should call 1-877-486-2048.

Note: You may lose your prescription drug coverage if you move from a Medicare Advantage Plan that has drug coverage to a Medicare Advantage Plan that doesn't. You will have to wait until the next open enrollment period to get drug coverage, and you may have to pay a late enrollment penalty. See page 90.

Blue words in the text are defined on pages 141–144.

How Do You Join?

If you choose to join a Medicare Advantage Plan, you may be able to join by doing the following:

- Enrolling on the plan's Web site or on www.medicare.gov.
- Completing a paper application.
- Calling the plan.
- Calling 1-800-MEDICARE (1-800-633-4227). TTY users should call 1-877-486-2048.

When you join a Medicare Advantage Plan, you will have to provide your Medicare number and the date your Part A and/or Part B coverage started. This information is on your Medicare card.

Medicare Advantage Plans aren't allowed to call you to enroll you in a plan. Also, plans should never ask you for financial information, including credit card or bank account numbers, over the phone. Call 1-800-MEDICARE to report a plan that does this. Don't give your personal information to anyone who calls you to enroll in a plan.

How Do You Switch?

Follow these steps if you're already in a Medicare Advantage Plan and want to switch:

- To switch to a new Medicare Advantage Plan, simply join the plan you choose during one of the enrollment periods explained on pages 78–79. You will be disenrolled automatically from your old plan when your new plan's coverage begins.

- To switch to Original Medicare, contact your current plan, or call 1-800-MEDICARE (1-800-633-4227). TTY users should call 1-877-486-2048. Unless you have other drug coverage, you should carefully consider Medicare prescription drug coverage (Part D). You may also want to consider a Medicare Supplement Insurance (Medigap) policy. See pages 66–69 for more information about buying a Medigap policy.

For more information on joining, dropping, and switching plans, visit www.medicare.gov/publications to view the fact sheet "Understanding Medicare Enrollment Periods." You can also call 1-800-MEDICARE to find out if a copy can be mailed to you.

No one should call you or come to your home uninvited to sell Medicare products. See pages 116–119 for more information about how to protect yourself from identity theft and fraud. If you believe a plan has misled you, call 1-800-MEDICARE.

Blue words in the text are defined on pages 141–144.

Other Medicare Health Plans

Some types of Medicare health plans that provide health care coverage aren't Medicare Advantage Plans but are still part of Medicare. Some of these plans provide Part A (Hospital Insurance) and Part B (Medical Insurance) coverage, while most others provide only Part B coverage. In addition, some also provide Part D prescription drug coverage. These plans have some of the same rules as Medicare Advantage Plans. Some of these rules are explained briefly below and on the next page. However, each type of plan has special rules and exceptions, so you should contact any plans you're interested in to get more details.

Medicare Cost Plans

Medicare Cost Plans are a type of Medicare health plan available in certain areas of the country. Here's what you should know about Medicare Cost Plans:

- You can join even if you only have Part B.
- If you have Part A and Part B and go to a non-network provider, the services are covered under Original Medicare. You would pay the Part A and Part B coinsurance and deductibles.
- You can join anytime the plan is accepting new members.
- You can leave anytime and return to Original Medicare.
- You can either get your Medicare prescription drug coverage from the plan (if offered), or you can join a Medicare Prescription Drug Plan. **Note:** You can add or drop Medicare prescription drug coverage only at certain times. See page 85.

There is another type of Medicare Cost Plan that only provides coverage for Part B services. These plans never include Part D. Part A services are covered through Original Medicare. These plans are either sponsored by employer or union group health plans or offered by companies that don't provide Part A services.

For more information about Medicare Cost Plans, contact the plans you're interested in. You can also visit the Medicare Plan Finder at www.medicare.gov/find-a-plan. Your State Health Insurance Assistance Program (SHIP) can also give you more information. See pages 137–140 for the phone number.

Blue words in the text are defined on pages 141–144.

Other Medicare Health Plans (continued)

Demonstrations/Pilot Programs

Demonstrations and pilot programs (also called "research studies") are special projects that test and measure the effect of potential changes in Medicare coverage, payment, and quality of care. Usually, they operate only for a limited time for a specific group of people and/or are offered only in specific areas. Check with the demonstration or pilot program for more information about how it works.

To find out about current Medicare demonstrations and pilot programs, call 1-800-MEDICARE (1-800-633-4227), and say "Agent." TTY users should call 1-877-486-2048.

Programs of All-Inclusive Care for the Elderly (PACE)

PACE is a Medicare and Medicaid program offered in many states that allows people who otherwise need a nursing home-level of care to remain in the community.

To qualify for PACE, you must meet the following conditions:
- You're 55 or older.
- You live in the service area of a PACE organization.
- You're certified by your state as needing a nursing home-level of care.
- At the time you join, you're able to live safely in the community with the help of PACE services.

PACE provides coverage for prescription drugs, doctor or other health care provider visits, transportation, home care, hospital visits, and even nursing home stays whenever necessary. If you have Medicaid, you won't have to pay a monthly premium for the long-term care portion of the PACE benefit. If you have Medicare but not Medicaid, you will be charged a monthly premium to cover the long-term care portion of the PACE benefit and a premium for Medicare Part D drugs. However, in PACE there is never a deductible or copayment for any drug, service, or care approved by the PACE team of health care professionals.

Call your State Medical Assistance (Medicaid) office to find out if you're eligible and if there is a PACE site near you, or visit www.pace4you.org. You can also visit www.medicare.gov/publications to view the fact sheet "Quick Facts about Programs of All-Inclusive Care for the Elderly (PACE)." You can call 1-800-MEDICARE to find out if a copy can be mailed to you.

Medicare Prescription Drug Coverage (Part D)

Medicare offers prescription drug coverage to everyone with Medicare. Even if you don't take a lot of prescriptions now, it's very important for you to consider joining a Medicare drug plan. If you decide not to join a Medicare drug plan when you're first eligible, and you don't have other creditable prescription drug coverage, or you don't get Extra Help, you will likely pay a late enrollment penalty. See pages 90–91. To get Medicare prescription drug coverage, you must join a plan run by an insurance company or other private company approved by Medicare. Each plan can vary in cost and specific drugs covered.

There are two ways to get Medicare prescription drug coverage:

1. **Medicare Prescription Drug Plans.** These plans (sometimes called "PDPs") add drug coverage to Original Medicare, some Medicare Cost Plans, some Medicare Private Fee-for-Service (PFFS) Plans, and Medicare Medical Savings Account (MSA) Plans.

2. **Medicare Advantage Plans (like an HMO or PPO) or other** Medicare health plans **that offer Medicare prescription drug coverage.** You get all of your Part A and Part B coverage, and prescription drug coverage (Part D), through these plans. Medicare Advantage Plans with prescription drug coverage are sometimes called "MA-PDs." You must have Part A and Part B to join a Medicare Advantage Plan.

In either case, you must live in the service area **of the Medicare drug plan you want to join. Both types of plans are called "Medicare drug plans" in this handbook.**

If you have employer or union coverage, call your benefits administrator before you make any changes, or before you sign up for any other coverage. If you drop your employer or union coverage, you may not be able to get it back. You also may not be able to drop your employer or union **drug** coverage without also dropping your employer or union **health** (doctor and hospital) coverage. If you drop coverage for yourself, you may also have to drop coverage for your spouse and dependants. If you want to know how Medicare prescription drug coverage works with other drug coverage you may have, see pages 95–96.

Join, Switch, or Drop a Medicare Drug Plan

- **When you're first eligible for Medicare,** you can join during the 7-month period that begins 3 months before the month you turn 65, includes the month you turn 65, and ends 3 months after the month you turn 65.

- **If you get Medicare due to a disability,** you can join during the 7-month period that begins 3 months before your 25th month of disability and ends 3 months after your 25th month of disability. You will have another chance to join during the 7-month period that begins 3 months before the month you turn 65 and ends 3 months after the month you turn 65.

- **NEW—Between October 15–December 7, anyone can join, switch, or drop a Medicare drug plan.** The change will take effect on January 1 as long as the plan gets your request by December 7.

- **Anytime, if you qualify for** Extra Help.

You generally must stay enrolled for the calendar year. However, in certain situations like the following, you may be able to join, switch, or drop Medicare drug plans at other times:

- If you move out of your plan's service area
- If you lose other creditable prescription drug coverage
- If you live in an institution (like a nursing home)

Call your State Health Insurance Assistance Program (SHIP) for more information. See pages 137–140 for the phone number. You can also call 1-800-MEDICARE (1-800-633-4227). TTY users should call 1-877-486-2048.

Note: If you have limited income and resources, you may qualify for Extra Help to pay for Medicare prescription drug coverage. You may also be able to get help from your state. See pages 98–104.

NEW—5-Star Special Enrollment Period
Starting December 8, 2011, you can switch to a 5-star Medicare Prescription Drug Plan **at any time during the year**. The overall plan star ratings are available at www.medicare.gov/find-a-plan. See page 79 for more information.

- You can only switch to a 5-star Medicare Prescription Drug Plan if one is available in your area.

- You can only use this period to switch to a 5-star plan one time each year.

Visit the Medicare Plan Finder at www.medicare.gov/find-a-plan to search for plans. For more information about overall plan ratings, visit www.medicare.gov/publications to view the fact sheet "Use Medicare's Information on Quality to Help You Compare Plans." You can also call 1-800-MEDICARE.

Blue words in the text are defined on pages 141–144.

How Do You Join?

Once you choose a Medicare drug plan, you may be able to join by doing the following:

- Enrolling on the plan's Web site or on www.medicare.gov.
- Completing a paper application.
- Calling the plan.
- Calling 1-800-MEDICARE (1-800-633-4227). TTY users should call 1-877-486-2048.

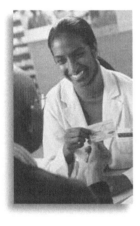

When you join a Medicare drug plan, you will have to provide your Medicare number and the date your Part A and/or Part B coverage started. This information is on your Medicare card.

Note: Medicare drug plans aren't allowed to call you to enroll you in a plan. Call 1-800-MEDICARE to report a plan that does this. Don't give your personal information to anyone who calls you to enroll in a plan.

How Do You Switch?

You can switch to a new Medicare drug plan simply by joining another drug plan during one of the times listed on page 85. **You don't need to cancel your old Medicare drug plan or send them anything**. Your old Medicare drug plan coverage will end when your new drug plan begins. You should get a letter from your new Medicare drug plan telling you when your coverage begins.

How Do You Drop a Medicare Drug Plan?

If you want to drop your Medicare drug plan and you don't want to join a new plan, you can do so during one of the times listed on page 85. You can disenroll by calling 1-800-MEDICARE. You can also send a letter to the plan to tell them you want to disenroll. If you drop your plan and want to join another Medicare drug plan later, you have to wait for an enrollment period. You may have to pay a late enrollment penalty. See pages 90–91.

If your Medicare Advantage Plan includes prescription drug coverage and you join a Medicare Prescription Drug Plan, you will be disenrolled from your Medicare Advantage Plan and returned to Original Medicare.

For more information, visit www.medicare.gov/publications to view the fact sheet "Understanding Medicare Enrollment Periods." You can also call 1-800-MEDICARE to find out if a copy can be mailed to you.

What You Pay

Below and continued on the next page are descriptions of the payments you make throughout the year in a Medicare drug plan. **Your actual drug plan costs will vary** depending on the following:

- The prescriptions you use and whether your plan covers them
- The plan you choose
- Whether you go to a pharmacy in your plan's network
- Whether your drugs are on your plan's formulary (drug list)
- Whether you get Extra Help paying your Part D costs

Monthly Premium

Most drug plans charge a monthly fee that varies by plan. You pay this in addition to the Part B premium. If you belong to a Medicare Advantage Plan (like an HMO or PPO) or a Medicare Cost Plan that includes Medicare prescription drug coverage, the monthly premium you pay to your plan may include an amount for prescription drug coverage.

Note: Contact your drug plan (not Social Security) if you want your premium deducted from your monthly Social Security payment. Your first deduction will usually take 3 months to start, and 3 months of premiums will likely be deducted at once. After that, only one premium will be deducted each month. You may also see a delay in premiums being withheld if you switch plans. If you want to stop premium deductions and get billed directly, contact your drug plan.

What you pay for Part D coverage could be higher based on your income. This includes Part D coverage you get from a Medicare Prescription Drug Plan, a Medicare Advantage Plan, a Medicare Cost Plan, or employer group Medicare Advantage Plan that includes Medicare prescription drug coverage.
If your modified adjusted gross income as reported on your IRS tax return from 2 years ago (the most recent tax return information provided to Social Security by the IRS) is above a certain limit, you will pay an extra amount in addition to your plan premium. Usually, the extra amount will be deducted from your Social Security check. If you have to pay an extra amount and you disagree (for example, you have a life event that lowers your income), call Social Security at 1-800-772-1213. TTY users should call 1-800-325-0778. For more information, visit www.socialsecurity.gov.

Yearly Deductible

The amount you must pay before your drug plan begins to pay its share of your covered drugs. Some drug plans don't have a deductible.

Copayments or Coinsurance

Amounts you pay for your covered prescriptions after the deductible (if the plan has one). You pay your share and your drug plan pays its share for covered drugs.

Blue words in the text are defined on pages 141–144.

What You Pay (continued)

Coverage Gap

Most Medicare drug plans have a coverage gap (also called the "donut hole"). This means that there is a temporary limit on what the drug plan will cover for drugs. The coverage gap begins after you and your drug plan have spent a certain amount for covered drugs. Once you enter the coverage gap, you get a 50% discount on covered brand name drugs and pay 86% of the plan's cost for covered generic drugs until you reach the end of the coverage gap. Not everyone will enter the coverage gap. The following items all count toward you getting out of the coverage gap:

- Your yearly deductible, coinsurance, and copayments
- The discount you get on brand-name drugs in the coverage gap
- What you pay in the coverage gap

The drug plan premium and what you pay for drugs that aren't covered **don't** count toward getting you out of the coverage gap.

There are plans that offer additional coverage during the gap, like for generic drugs. However, plans with additional gap coverage may charge a higher monthly premium. Check with the drug plan first to see if your drugs would be covered during the gap.

In addition to the 50% discount on covered brand-name prescription drugs, there will be increasing savings for you in the coverage gap each year until the gap closes in 2020. Talk to your doctor or other health care provider to make sure that you're taking the lowest cost drug available that works for you. For more information, visit www.medicare.gov/publications to view the fact sheet "Closing the Coverage Gap—Medicare Prescription Drugs Are Becoming More Affordable." You can also call 1-800-MEDICARE (1-800-633-4227) to find out if a copy can be mailed to you. TTY users should call 1-877-486-2048.

Catastrophic Coverage

Once you get out of the coverage gap, you automatically get "catastrophic coverage." Catastrophic coverage assures that you only pay a small coinsurance amount or copayment for covered drugs for the rest of the year.

Note: If you get Extra Help, some of these costs won't apply to you. See page 98.

Blue words in the text are defined on pages 141–144.

What You Pay (continued)

The example below shows costs for covered drugs in 2012 for a plan that has a coverage gap.

Ms. Smith joins the ABC Prescription Drug Plan. Her coverage begins on January 1, 2012. She doesn't get Extra Help and uses her Medicare drug plan membership card when she buys prescriptions.

Monthly Premium—Ms. Smith pays a monthly premium throughout the year.			
1. Yearly Deductible ➡	**2. Copayment or Coinsurance (What you pay at the pharmacy)** ➡	**3. Coverage Gap** ➡	**4. Catastrophic Coverage** ➡
Ms. Smith pays the first $320 of her drug costs before her plan starts to pay its share.	Ms. Smith pays a copayment, and her plan pays its share for each covered drug until their **combined** amount (plus the deductible) reaches $2,930.	Once Ms. Smith and her plan have spent $2,930 for covered drugs, she is in the coverage gap. In 2012, she gets a 50% discount on covered brand-name prescription drugs and she pays 86% of the plan's cost for covered generic drugs. What she pays (and the 50% discount paid by the drug company) counts as out-of-pocket spending, and helps her get out of the coverage gap.	Once Ms. Smith has spent $4,700 out-of-pocket for the year, her coverage gap ends. Now she only pays a small coinsurance or copayment for each drug until the end of the year.

To get specific Medicare drug plan costs, call the plans you're interested in. You can also visit the Medicare Plan Finder at www.medicare.gov/find-a-plan, or call 1-800-MEDICARE (1-800-633-4227). TTY users should call 1-877-486-2048. For help comparing plan costs, contact your State Health Insurance Assistance Program (SHIP). See pages 137–140 for the phone number.

What is the Part D Late Enrollment Penalty?

The late enrollment penalty is an amount that's added to your Part D premium. You may owe a late enrollment penalty if at any time after your initial enrollment period is over, there is a period of 63 or more days in a row when you don't have Part D or other creditable prescription drug coverage.

Note: If you get Extra Help, you don't pay a late enrollment penalty.

Here are a few ways to avoid paying a penalty:

- **Join a Medicare drug plan when you're first eligible.** You won't have to pay a penalty, even if you've never had prescription drug coverage before.

- **Don't go 63 days or more in a row without a Medicare drug plan or other creditable coverage.** Creditable prescription drug coverage could include drug coverage from a current or former employer or union, TRICARE, Indian Health Service, the Department of Veterans Affairs, or health insurance coverage. Your plan must tell you each year if your drug coverage is creditable coverage. This information may be sent to you in a letter or included in a newsletter from the plan. Keep this information, because you may need it if you join a Medicare drug plan later.

- **Tell your plan about any drug coverage you had if they ask about it.** When you join a Medicare drug plan, and the plan believes you went at least 63 days in a row without other creditable prescription drug coverage, the plan will send you a letter. The letter will include a form asking about any drug coverage you had. Complete the form and return it to your drug plan. If you don't tell the plan about your creditable prescription drug coverage, you may have to pay a penalty.

Blue words in the text are defined on pages 141–144.

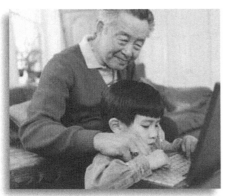

How Much More Will You Pay?

The cost of the late enrollment penalty depends on how long you didn't have creditable prescription drug coverage. Currently, the late enrollment penalty is calculated by multiplying 1% of the "national base beneficiary premium" ($32.34 in 2011) times the number of full, uncovered months that you were eligible but didn't join a Medicare drug plan and went without other creditable prescription drug coverage. The final amount is rounded to the nearest $.10 and added to your monthly premium. Since the "national base beneficiary premium" may increase each year, the penalty amount may also increase every year. You may have to pay this penalty for as long as you have a Medicare drug plan.

> **Example:** Mrs. Jones didn't join when she was first eligible—by May 15, 2007. She joined a Medicare drug plan with an effective date of January 1, 2011. Since Mrs. Jones didn't join when she was first eligible and went without other creditable drug coverage for 43 months (June 2007–December 2010), she will be charged a monthly penalty of $13.90 in 2011 ($32.34 X .01 = $.3234 X 43 = $13.90) in addition to her plan's monthly premium.

After you join a Medicare drug plan, the plan will tell you if you owe a penalty, and what your premium will be.

If You Don't Agree With Your Penalty

If you don't agree with your late enrollment penalty, you can ask Medicare for a review or reconsideration. You will need to fill out a reconsideration request form (that your Medicare drug plan will send you), and you will have the chance to provide proof that supports your case, such as information about previous creditable prescription drug coverage. If you need help, call your Medicare plan. You can also contact your State Health Insurance Assistance Program (SHIP). See pages 137–140 for the phone number.

Important Drug Coverage Rules

The following information can help answer common questions as you begin to use your coverage.

To Fill a Prescription Before You Get Your Membership Card

You should get a welcome package with your membership card within 5 weeks after the plan gets your completed application. If you need to go to the pharmacy before your membership card arrives, you can use any of the following as proof of membership:

- A letter from the plan that includes your membership information. You should get this letter within 2 weeks after the plan gets your completed application.

- An enrollment confirmation number that you got from the plan, the plan name, and phone number.

- A temporary card that you may be able to print from MyMedicare.gov. Visit www.MyMedicare.gov for more information, or see page 130.

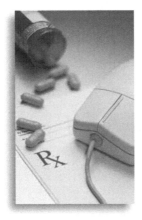

If you don't have any of the items listed above, your pharmacist may be able to get your drug plan information if you provide your Medicare number or the last 4 digits of your Social Security number. If your pharmacist can't get your drug plan information, you may have to pay out-of-pocket for your prescriptions. **If you do, save the receipts and contact your plan to get your money back**.

If you qualify for Extra Help, see pages 98–101 for more information about what you can use as proof of Extra Help.

Note: Every month that you fill a prescription, your drug plan mails you an Explanation of Benefits (EOB) notice. This notice gives you a summary of your prescription drug claims and your costs. Review your notice and check it for mistakes. Contact your plan if you have questions or find mistakes. If you suspect fraud, call the Medicare Drug Integrity Contractor (MEDIC) at 1-877-7SAFERX (1-877-772-3379). See page 116 for more information about the MEDIC.

Important Drug Coverage Rules (continued)

What's Covered?

Information about a plan's list of covered drugs (called a formulary) isn't included in this handbook because each plan has its own formulary. Many Medicare drug plans place drugs into different "tiers" on their formularies. Drugs in each tier have a different cost. For example, a drug in a lower tier will generally cost you less than a drug in a higher tier. In some cases, if your drug is on a higher tier and your prescriber (your doctor or other health care provider who is legally allowed to write prescriptions) thinks you need that drug instead of a similar drug on a lower tier, you or your prescriber can ask your plan for an exception to get a lower copayment.

Contact the plan for its current formulary, or visit the plan's Web site. Visit the Medicare Plan Finder at www.medicare.gov/find-a-plan to get phone numbers for the plans in your area. You can also call 1-800-MEDICARE (1-800-633-4227). TTY users should call 1-877-486-2048. Your plan will notify you of any formulary changes.

Note: Medicare drug plans must cover all commercially-available vaccines (like the shingles vaccine) when medically necessary to prevent illness, except for vaccines covered under Part B.

If you're in a Medicare drug plan and you have complex health needs, you may be eligible to participate in a Medication Therapy Management (MTM) program. These programs help you and your doctor make sure that your medications are working. MTM programs include a free discussion and review of all of your medications by a pharmacist or other health professional to help you use them safely. You will get a summary of this discussion to help you get the most benefit from your medications. You can have this summary available when you talk with your doctors or other health care providers. If you take many medications for more than one chronic health condition, contact your drug plan to see if you're eligible.

Blue words in the text are defined on pages 141–144.

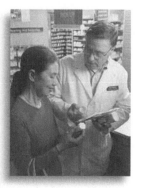

Important Drug Coverage Rules (continued)

Plans may have the following coverage rules:

- **Prior authorization**—You and/or your prescriber must contact the drug plan before you can fill certain prescriptions. Your prescriber may need to show that the drug is medically necessary for the plan to cover it.

- **Quantity limits**—Limits on how much medication you can get at a time.

- **Step therapy**—You must try one or more similar, lower cost drugs before the plan will cover the prescribed drug.

If you or your prescriber believe that one of these coverage rules should be waived, you can ask for an exception. See pages 110–111.

Blue words in the text are defined on pages 141–144.

In most cases, the prescription drugs (sometimes called "self-administered drugs" or drugs you would usually take on your own) you get in an outpatient setting, like an emergency department, or during observation services aren't covered by Part B. Your Medicare drug plan may cover these drugs under certain circumstances. You will likely need to pay out-of-pocket for these drugs and submit a claim to your drug plan for a refund. Or, if you get a bill for self-administered drugs you got in a doctor's office, call your Medicare drug plan (Part D) for more information. Visit www.medicare.gov/publications to view the fact sheet, "How Medicare Covers Self-Administered Drugs Given in Hospital Outpatient Settings." You can also call 1-800-MEDICARE (1-800-633-4227) to find out if a copy can be mailed to you. TTY users should call 1-877-486-2048.

Other Private Insurance

The charts on the next two pages provide information about how other insurance you have works with, or is affected by, Medicare prescription drug coverage (Part D).

Employer or Union Health Coverage—Health coverage from your, your spouse's, or other family member's current or former employer or union. If you have prescription drug coverage based on your current or previous employment, your employer or union will notify you each year to let you know if your prescription drug coverage is creditable. **Keep the information you get**. Call your benefits administrator for more information before making any changes to your coverage. **Note:** If you join a Medicare drug plan, you, your spouse, or your dependants may lose your employer or union health coverage.

COBRA—A Federal law that may allow you to temporarily keep employer or union health coverage after the employment ends or after you lose coverage as a dependent of the covered employee. As explained on pages 24–25, there may be reasons why you should take Part B instead of, or in addition to, COBRA. However, if you take COBRA and it includes creditable prescription drug coverage, you will have a special enrollment period to join a Medicare drug plan without paying a penalty when the COBRA coverage ends. Talk with your State Health Insurance Assistance Program (SHIP) to see if COBRA is a good choice for you. See pages 137–140 for the phone number.

Medicare Supplement Insurance (Medigap) Policy with Prescription Drug Coverage—It may be to your advantage to join a Medicare drug plan because most Medigap drug coverage isn't creditable and you may pay more if you join a drug plan later. See pages 90–91. Medigap policies can no longer be sold with prescription drug coverage, but if you have drug coverage under a current Medigap policy, you can keep it. If you join a Medicare drug plan, your Medigap insurance company must remove the prescription drug coverage under your Medigap policy and adjust your premiums. Call your Medigap insurance company for more information.

Note: Keep any creditable prescription drug coverage information you get from your plan. You may need it if you decide to join a Medicare drug plan later. Don't send creditable coverage letters/certificates to Medicare.

Other Government Insurance

The types of insurance listed on this page are all considered creditable prescription drug coverage. If you have one of these types of insurance, in most cases, it will be to your advantage to keep your current coverage.

Blue words in the text are defined on pages 141–144.

Federal Employee Health Benefits (FEHB) Program—Health coverage for current and retired Federal employees and covered family members. FEHB plans usually include prescription drug coverage, so you don't need to join a Medicare drug plan. However, if you decide to join a Medicare drug plan, you can keep your FEHB plan, and your plan will let you know who pays first. For more information, contact the Office of Personnel Management at 1-888-767-6738, or visit www.opm.gov/insure. TTY users should call 1-800-878-5707. You can also call your plan if you have questions.

Veterans' Benefits—Health coverage for veterans and people who have served in the U.S. military. You may be able to get prescription drug coverage through the U.S. Department of Veterans Affairs (VA) program. You may join a Medicare drug plan, but if you do, you can't use both types of coverage for the same prescription at the same time. For more information, call the VA at 1-800-827-1000, or visit www.va.gov. TTY users should call 1-800-829-4833.

TRICARE (Military Health Benefits)—Health care plan for active-duty service members, retirees, and their families. **Most people with TRICARE who are entitled to Part A must have Part B to keep TRICARE prescription drug benefits**. If you have TRICARE, you don't need to join a Medicare Prescription Drug Plan. However, if you do, your Medicare drug plan pays first, and TRICARE pays second. If you join a Medicare Advantage Plan (like an HMO or PPO) with prescription drug coverage, your Medicare Advantage Plan and TRICARE may coordinate their benefits if your Medicare Advantage Plan network pharmacy is also a TRICARE network pharmacy. For more information, call the TRICARE Pharmacy Program at 1-877-363-1303, or visit www.tricare.mil/mybenefit. TTY users should call 1-877-540-6261.

Indian Health Services—Health care services for American Indians and Alaska Natives. Many Indian health facilities participate in the Medicare prescription drug program. If you get prescription drugs through an Indian health facility, you will continue to get drugs at no cost to you and your coverage won't be interrupted. Joining a Medicare drug plan may help your Indian health facility because the drug plan pays the Indian health facility for the cost of your prescriptions. Talk to your local Indian health benefits coordinator who can help you choose a plan that meets your needs and tell you how Medicare works with the Indian health care system.

Get Help Paying Your Health and Prescription Drug Costs

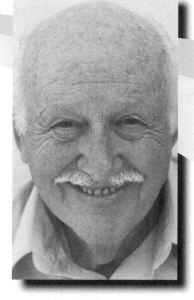

Section 4 includes information about the following:

Keep all information you get from Medicare, Social Security, your Medicare plan, Medicare Supplement Insurer, or employer or union. This may include notices of award or denial, Annual Notices of Change, notices of creditable prescription drug coverage, or Medicare Summary Notices. You may need these documents to apply for the programs explained in this section. Also keep copies of all applications you submit.

Programs for People with Limited Income and Resources

If you have limited income and resources, you might qualify for help to pay for some health care and prescription drug costs.

Extra Help Paying for Medicare Prescription Drug Coverage (Part D)

Extra Help is a Medicare program to help people with limited income and resources pay Medicare prescription drug costs. You may qualify for Extra Help, also called the low-income subsidy (LIS) if your yearly income and resources are below the following limits in 2011:

- Single person—Income less than $16,335 and resources less than $12,640

- Married person living with a spouse and no other dependants— Income less than $22,065 and resources less than $25,260

These amounts may change in 2012. You may qualify even if you have a higher income (like if you still work, live in Alaska or Hawaii, or have dependants living with you). Resources include money in a checking or savings account, stocks, bonds, mutual funds, and Individual Retirement Accounts (IRAs). Resources **don't** include your home, car, household items, burial plot, up to $1,500 for burial expenses (per person), or life insurance policies.

If you qualify for Extra Help and join a Medicare drug plan, you will get the following:

- Help paying your Medicare drug plan's monthly premium, yearly deductible, coinsurance, and copayments

- No coverage gap

- No late enrollment penalty

You **automatically** qualify for Extra Help if you have Medicare and meet one of these conditions:

- You have full Medicaid coverage

- You get help from your state Medicaid program paying your Part B premiums (in a Medicare Savings Program)

- You get Supplemental Security Income (SSI) benefits

Blue words in the text are defined on pages 141–144.

Extra Help Paying for Medicare Prescription Drug Coverage (Part D) (continued)

To let you know you automatically qualify for Extra Help, Medicare will mail you a purple letter that you should keep for your records. You don't need to apply for Extra Help if you get this letter.

- If you aren't already in a Medicare drug plan, you must join one to use this Extra Help.
- If you don't join a Medicare drug plan, Medicare may enroll you in one. If Medicare enrolls you in a plan, you will get a yellow or green letter letting you know when your coverage begins.
- Different plans cover different drugs. Check to see if the plan you're enrolled in covers the drugs you use and if you can go to the pharmacies you want. Compare with other plans in your area.
- If you're getting Extra Help, you can switch to another Medicare drug plan anytime. Your new coverage will be effective the first day of the next month.
- If you have Medicaid and live in certain institutions (like a nursing home) or get home and community-based services (see page 123), you pay nothing for your covered prescription drugs.

If you don't want to join a Medicare drug plan (for example, because you want only your employer or union coverage), call the plan listed in your letter, or call 1-800-MEDICARE (1-800-633-4227). TTY users should call 1-877-486-2048. Tell them you don't want to be in a Medicare drug plan (you want to "opt out"). If you continue to qualify for Extra Help or if your employer or union coverage is creditable prescription drug coverage, you won't have to pay a penalty if you join later.

If you have employer or union coverage and you join a Medicare drug plan, you may lose your employer or union coverage even if you qualify for Extra Help. Call your employer's benefits administrator for more information before you join.

Extra Help Paying for Medicare Prescription Drug Coverage (Part D) (continued)

If you didn't automatically qualify for Extra Help, you can apply:

- Visit www.socialsecurity.gov/i1020 to apply online.
- Call Social Security at 1-800-772-1213 to apply for Extra Help by phone or to get a paper application. TTY users should call 1-800-325-0778.
- Visit your State Medical Assistance (Medicaid) office. Visit www.medicare.gov/contacts or call 1-800-MEDICARE (1-800-633-4227) to get the phone number. TTY users should call 1-877-486-2048.

Note: You can apply for Extra Help at anytime. With your consent, Social Security will forward information to the Medicaid office in your state to start an application for a Medicare Savings Program. See page 102.

Drug costs in 2012 for most people who qualify will be no more than $2.60 for each generic drug and $6.50 for each brand name drug. Look on the Extra Help letters you get, or contact your plan to find out your exact costs.

To get answers to your questions about Extra Help and help choosing a plan, call your State Health Insurance Assistance Program (SHIP). See pages 137–140 for the phone number. You can also call 1-800-MEDICARE.

Paying the Right Amount

Medicare gets information from your state or Social Security that tells whether you qualify for Extra Help. If Medicare doesn't have the right information, you may be paying the wrong amount for your prescription drug coverage.

If you automatically qualify for Extra Help, you can show your drug plan the colored letter you got from Medicare as proof that you qualify. If you applied for Extra Help, you can show your "Notice of Award" from Social Security as proof that you qualify.

You can also give your plan **any** of the documents listed on the next page (also called "Best Available Evidence") as proof that you qualify for Extra Help. Your plan must accept these documents. Each item must show that you were eligible for Medicaid during a month after June of 2011.

Blue words in the text are defined on pages 141–144.

Extra Help Paying for Medicare Prescription Drug Coverage (Part D) (continued)

Paying the Right Amount (continued)

Proof You Have Medicaid and Live in an Institution or Get Home and Community-based Services	Other Proof You Have Medicaid
■ A bill from the institution (like a nursing home) or a copy of a state document showing Medicaid payment to the institution for at least a month ■ A print-out from your state's Medicaid system showing that you lived in the institution for at least a month ■ A document from your state that shows you have Medicaid and are getting home and community-based services	■ A copy of your Medicaid card (if you have one) ■ A copy of a state document that shows you have Medicaid ■ A print-out from a state electronic enrollment file or from your state's Medicaid system that shows you have Medicaid ■ Any other document from your state that shows you have Medicaid

If you aren't already enrolled in a Medicare drug plan and paid for prescriptions since you qualified for Extra Help, you may be able to get back part of what you paid. **Keep your receipts**, and call Medicare's Limited Income Newly Eligible Transition (NET) Program at 1-800-783-1307 for more information. TTY users should call 1-877-801-0369.

For more information, visit www.medicare.gov/publications to view the fact sheet "If You Get Extra Help, Make Sure You're Paying the Right Amount." You can also call 1-800-MEDICARE (1-800-633-4227) to find out if a copy can be mailed to you. TTY users should call 1-877-486-2048.

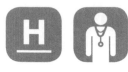

Medicare Savings Programs (Help with Medicare Costs)

States have programs that pay Medicare premiums and, in some cases, may also pay Part A and Part B deductibles, coinsurance, and copayments. These programs help people with Medicare who have limited income and resources. The names of these programs and how they work may vary by state.

In most cases, to qualify for a Medicare Savings Program, you must meet all of these conditions:

- Have Part A.
- Have monthly income less than $1,246 and resources less than $6,680—single person.
- Have monthly income less than $1,675 and resources less than $10,020—married and living together.

Note: These amounts may change each year. Many states figure your income and resources differently, so you may qualify in your state even if your income or resources are higher than the amounts listed above. If you have a disability and are working, you may qualify even if your income is higher. Resources include money in a checking or savings account, stocks, bonds, mutual funds, and Individual Retirement Accounts (IRAs). Resources **don't** include your home, car, burial plot, burial expenses up to your state's limit, furniture, or other household items. Some states don't have any limits on resources.

For More Information

- Call or visit your State Medical Assistance (Medicaid) office, and ask for information on Medicare Savings Programs. Call if you think you qualify for any of these programs, even if you aren't sure. To get the phone number for your state visit www.medicare.gov/contacts. You can also call 1-800-MEDICARE (1-800-633-4227), and say "Medicaid." TTY users should call 1-877-486-2048.

- Visit www.medicare.gov/publications to view the brochure "Get Help With Your Medicare Costs: Getting Started." You can also call 1-800-MEDICARE to find out if a copy can be mailed to you.

- Contact your State Health Insurance Assistance Program (SHIP). See pages 137–140 for the phone number.

Blue words in the text are defined on pages 141–144.

Medicaid

Medicaid is a joint Federal and state program that helps pay medical costs if you have limited income and resources and meet other requirements. Some people qualify for both Medicare and Medicaid and are called "dual eligibles."

- If you have Medicare and full Medicaid coverage, most of your health care costs are covered. You can get your Medicare coverage through Original Medicare or a Medicare Advantage Plan (like an HMO or PPO).

- If you have Medicare and full Medicaid, Medicare covers your prescription drugs. Medicaid may still cover some drugs and other care that Medicare doesn't cover.

- People with Medicaid may get coverage for services that Medicare doesn't fully cover, such as nursing home care.

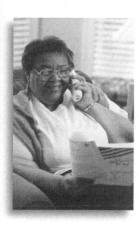

- Medicaid programs vary from state to state. They may also have different names, such as "Medical Assistance" or "Medi-Cal."

- Each state has different income and resource requirements.

- In some states, you may need Medicare to be eligible for Medicaid.

- Call your State Medical Assistance (Medicaid) office for more information and to see if you qualify. Visit www.medicare.gov/contacts. You can also call 1-800-MEDICARE (1-800-633-4227), and say "Medicaid" to get the phone number for your State Medical Assistance (Medicaid) office. TTY users should call 1-877-486-2048.

State Pharmacy Assistance Programs (SPAPs)

Many states have State Pharmacy Assistance Programs (SPAPs) that help certain people pay for prescription drugs based on financial need, age, or medical condition. Each SPAP makes its own rules on how to provide drug coverage to its members. To find out about the SPAP in your state, call your State Health Insurance Assistance Program (SHIP). See pages 137–140 for the phone number.

Pharmaceutical Assistance Programs (also called Patient Assistance Programs)

Many major drug manufacturers offer assistance programs for people with Medicare drug coverage who meet certain requirements.

Note: Visit www.medicare.gov/pap/index.asp to learn more about Pharmaceutical Assistance Programs.

Programs of All-Inclusive Care for the Elderly (PACE)

PACE is a Medicare and Medicaid program offered in many states that allows people who need a nursing home-level of care to remain in the community. See page 83 for more information.

Supplemental Security Income (SSI) Benefits

SSI is a cash benefit paid by Social Security to people with limited income and resources who are disabled, blind, or 65 or older. SSI benefits help people meet basic needs for food, clothing, and shelter. SSI benefits aren't the same as Social Security benefits.

You can visit www.socialsecurity.gov, and use the "Benefit Eligibility Screening Tool" to find out if you're eligible for SSI or other benefits. Call Social Security at 1-800-772-1213 or contact your local Social Security office for more information. TTY users should call 1-800-325-0778.

Note: People who live in Puerto Rico, the U.S. Virgin Islands, Guam, or American Samoa can't get SSI.

Programs for People Who Live in the U.S. Territories

There are programs in Puerto Rico, the U.S. Virgin Islands, Guam, the Northern Mariana Islands, and American Samoa to help people with limited income and resources pay their Medicare costs. This help isn't the same as the Extra Help described on pages 98–101. Programs vary in these areas. Call your local Medical Assistance (Medicaid) office to learn more, or call 1-800-MEDICARE (1-800-633-4227) and say "Medicaid" for more information. TTY users should call 1-877-486-2048.

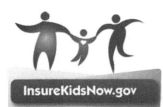

Children's Health Insurance Program

Do you have children or grandchildren who need health insurance? The Children's Health Insurance Program provides low cost health insurance coverage to children in families who earn too much income to qualify for Medicaid, but not enough to buy private health insurance.

Each state has its own program, with its own eligibility rules. Call 1-877-KIDS-NOW (1-877-543-7669), or visit www.insurekidsnow.gov for more information about the Children's Health Insurance Program.

Blue words in the text are defined on pages 141–144.

Protecting Yourself and Medicare

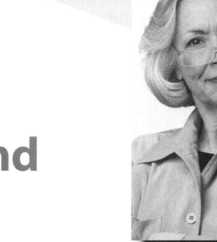

Section 5 includes information about the following:

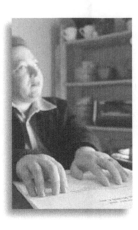

Your Medicare Rights

No matter what type of Medicare coverage you have, you have certain guaranteed rights. As a person with Medicare, you have the right to all of the following:

- Be treated with dignity and respect at all times

- Be protected from discrimination

- Have access to doctors, other health care providers, specialists, and hospitals

- Have your questions about Medicare answered

- Learn about your treatment choices and participate in treatment decisions

- Get information in a way you understand from Medicare, health care providers, and under certain circumstances, contractors

- Get emergency care when and where you need it

- Get a decision about health care payment or coverage of services, or prescription drug coverage

- Get a review (appeal) of certain decisions about health care payment, coverage of services, or prescription drug coverage

- File complaints (sometimes called grievances), including complaints about the quality of your care

- Have your personal and health information kept private

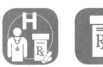

Your Rights if Your Plan Stops Participating in Medicare

Medicare health and prescription drug plans can decide not to participate in Medicare for the coming year. Plans that choose to leave Medicare entirely or in certain areas are said to be "non-renewing." In these cases, the plan will send you a letter about your options and your right to join another Medicare plan.

If you want to continue to have Medicare prescription drug coverage (Part D) or a Medicare Advantage Plan (like an HMO or PPO), you need to join a new plan for the coming year. If you join a new Medicare plan by December 31, you will have coverage as of January 1. If you don't join a new Medicare Advantage Plan by December 31, you will continue to have Medicare coverage through Original Medicare. If you don't join a Part D plan by that date, you will no longer have Medicare drug coverage.

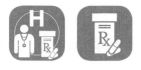

Your Rights if Your Plan Stops Participating in Medicare (continued)

If you didn't join a new plan by December 31, you will have until February 29, 2012, to choose and join a new Medicare plan.

- Generally, if you're in a Medicare health plan, you will automatically return to Original Medicare if you don't choose to join another Medicare health plan. You will also have the right to buy certain Medigap policies. If you return to Original Medicare, you can also join a Medicare Prescription Drug Plan.

- If you're in a Medicare Prescription Drug Plan, you will have the right to join another Medicare Prescription Drug Plan or a Medicare health plan with drug coverage. If you don't join a new plan, you won't have Medicare prescription drug coverage (Part D).

What is an Appeal?

An appeal is the action you can take if you disagree with a coverage or payment decision made by Medicare or your Medicare plan. You can appeal if Medicare or your plan denies one of the following:

- A request for a health care service, supply, item, or prescription drug that you think you should be able to get

- A request for payment for health care services, supplies, items, or prescription drugs you already got

- A request to change the amount you must pay for a prescription drug

You can also appeal if Medicare or your plan stops **providing or paying for all or part of** an item or service you think you still need.

If you decide to file an appeal, you can ask your doctor or other health care provider or supplier for any information that may help your case.

Blue words in the text are defined on pages 141–144.

How to File an Appeal

How you file an appeal depends on the type of Medicare coverage you have:

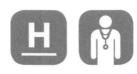

- If you have Original Medicare, do the following to file an appeal:

  1. Get the Medicare Summary Notice (MSN) that shows the item or service you're appealing. Your MSN is the notice you get every 3 months that lists all the services billed to Medicare and tells you if Medicare paid for the services. See page 61.

  2. Circle the item(s) you disagree with on the notice, and write an explanation on the notice of why you disagree. You can also write your explanation on a separate page and send it in with the notice.

  3. Sign, write your phone number, and provide your Medicare number on the notice. Keep a copy for your records.

  4. Send the notice, or a copy, to the Medicare contractor's address listed on the notice. You can also send any additional information you may have about your appeal.

  5. You must file the appeal within 120 days of the date you get the notice.

     Or you can use CMS Form 20027, and file it with the Medicare contractor at the address listed on the notice. To view or print this form, visit www.medicare.gov/medicareonlineforms, or call 1-800-MEDICARE (1-800-633-4227) for a copy of the form. TTY users should call 1-877-486-2048.

     You will generally get a decision from the Medicare contractor (either in a letter or an MSN) within 60 days after they get your request. If Medicare will cover the item(s), it will be listed on your next notice.

- If you have a Medicare plan, learn how to file an appeal by looking at the materials your plan sends you, calling your plan, or visiting www.medicare.gov/publications to view the booklet "Medicare Appeals." You can also call 1-800-MEDICARE to find out if a copy can be mailed to you.

In some cases, you can file a fast appeal. See materials from your plan and page 109.

Contact your State Health Insurance Assistance Program (SHIP) if you need help filing an appeal. See pages 137–140 for the phone number.

Blue words in the text are defined on pages 141–144.

Your Rights if You Think Your Services are Ending Too Soon

If you're getting Medicare services from a hospital, skilled nursing facility, home health agency, comprehensive outpatient rehabilitation facility, or hospice, and you think your Medicare-covered services are ending too soon, you can ask for a fast appeal. Your provider will give you a notice before your services end that will tell you how to ask for a fast appeal. You should read this notice carefully. If you don't get this notice, ask your provider for it. With a fast appeal, an independent reviewer, called a Quality Improvement Organization (QIO), will decide if your services should continue.

- You may ask your doctor or other health care provider for any information that may help your case if you decide to file a fast appeal.

- You must call your QIO to request a fast appeal no later than the time shown on the notice you get from your provider. Use the phone number for your QIO listed on your notice to request your appeal.

- If you miss the deadline, you still have appeal rights:
  - If you have Original Medicare, call your QIO.
  - If you're in a Medicare health plan, read your notice carefully and follow the instructions for filing an appeal with your plan. You can also call your plan.

Visit www.medicare.gov/contacts or call 1-800-MEDICARE (1-800-633-4227) to get the phone number for the QIO in your state. TTY users should call 1-877-486-2048.

Appealing Your Medicare Drug Plan's Decisions

If you have Medicare prescription drug coverage (Part D), you have the right to do all of the following (even before you buy your prescription):

- Get a written explanation (called a "coverage determination") from your Medicare drug plan. A coverage determination is the first decision made by your Medicare drug plan (not the pharmacy) about your prescription drug benefits. This includes whether a certain drug is covered, whether you have met all the requirements for getting a requested drug, and how much you're required to pay for a drug.

- Ask for an exception if you or your prescriber (your doctor or other health care provider who is legally allowed to write prescriptions) believes you need a drug that isn't on your plan's formulary.

- Ask for an exception if you or your prescriber believes that a coverage rule (such as prior authorization) should be waived.

- Ask for an exception if you think you should pay less for a higher tier (more expensive) drug because you or your prescriber believes you can't take any of the lower tier (less expensive) drugs for the same condition.

You or your prescriber must contact your plan to ask for a coverage determination, including an exception. If your network pharmacy can't fill a prescription as written, the pharmacist will give you a notice that explains how to contact your Medicare drug plan so you can make your request. If the pharmacist doesn't give you this notice, ask for it.

Appealing Your Medicare Drug Plan's Decisions (continued)

You or your prescriber may make a standard appeal request by phone or in writing, if you're asking for prescription drug benefits you haven't received yet. If you're asking to get paid back for prescription drugs you already bought, your plan can require you or your prescriber to make the standard request in writing.

You or your prescriber can call or write your plan for an expedited (fast) request. Your request will be expedited if you haven't received the prescription and your plan determines, or your prescriber tells your plan, that your life or health may be at risk by waiting.

Once your plan has received your request, it has 72 hours (for a standard request for coverage) or 24 hours (for an expedited request for coverage) to notify you of its decision.

If you're requesting an exception, your prescriber must provide a statement explaining the medical reason why the exception should be approved.

Appealing Your Medicare Drug Plan's Decisions (continued)

If you disagree with your Medicare drug plan's coverage determination, including an exception decision, you can appeal. The first level is appealing to your plan. Once your Medicare drug plan gets your appeal, it has 7 days (for a standard appeal) or 72 hours (for an expedited appeal) to notify you of its decision. If you disagree with the plan's decision, you can ask for an independent review of your case. The notice you get with the plan's decision will explain what you can do next.

You can get help filing an appeal from your State Health Insurance Assistance Program (SHIP). See pages 137–140 for the phone number.

If your plan doesn't respond to your request for a coverage determination including an exception, or an appeal, you can file a complaint (also called a grievance). Call your plan. You can also call 1-800-MEDICARE (1-800-633-4227). TTY users should call 1-877-486-2048.

For more information about the different levels of appeals in a Medicare drug plan, visit www.medicare.gov/publications to view the booklet "Medicare Appeals." You can also call 1-800-MEDICARE to find out if a copy can be mailed to you.

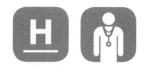

Advance Beneficiary Notice (ABN)

If you have Original Medicare, your health care provider or supplier may give you a notice called an "Advance Beneficiary Notice" (ABN).

- This notice says Medicare probably (or certainly) won't pay for some services in certain situations.

- You will be asked to choose whether to get the items or services listed on the ABN.

- If you choose to get the items or services listed on the ABN, you will have to pay if Medicare doesn't.

- You will be asked to sign the ABN to say that you have read and understood it.

- Doctors, other health care providers, and suppliers don't have to (but still may) give you an ABN for services that Medicare never covers. See page 54.

- An ABN isn't an official denial of coverage by Medicare. You could choose to get the items listed on the ABN and still ask your health care provider or supplier to submit the bill to Medicare or another insurer. If Medicare denies payment, you can still file an appeal. However, you will have to pay for the items or services if Medicare determines that the items or services aren't covered (and no other insurer is responsible for payment).

- You may get a Home Health ABN for other reasons, such as when your doctor or other health care provider makes changes to or reduces your home health care.

- You may get a Skilled Nursing Facility ABN when the facility believes Medicare will no longer cover your stay.

- If you should have received an ABN but didn't, in most cases your provider must pay you back what you paid for the item or service.

If you're in a Medicare plan, call your plan to find out if a service or item will be covered.

Blue words in the text are defined on pages 141–144.

For more information about ABNs, visit www.medicare.gov/publications to view the booklet "Medicare Appeals." You can also call 1-800-MEDICARE (1-800-633-4227) to find out if a copy can be mailed to you. TTY users should call 1-877-486-2048.

How Medicare Uses Your Personal Information

You have the right to have your personal and health information kept private. The next two pages describe how your information may be used and given out and explain how you can get this information.

Notice of Privacy Practices for Original Medicare
THIS NOTICE DESCRIBES HOW MEDICAL INFORMATION ABOUT YOU MAY BE USED AND DISCLOSED AND HOW YOU CAN GET ACCESS TO THIS INFORMATION. PLEASE REVIEW IT CAREFULLY.

By law, Medicare is required to protect the privacy of your personal medical information. Medicare is also required to give you this notice to tell you how Medicare may use and give out ("disclose") your personal medical information held by Medicare.

Medicare must use and give out your personal medical information to provide information to the following:

- To you or someone who has the legal right to act for you (your personal representative)
- To the Secretary of the Department of Health and Human Services, if necessary, to make sure your privacy is protected
- Where required by law

Medicare has the right to use and give out your personal medical information to pay for your health care and to operate the Medicare Program. Examples include the following:

- Companies that pay bills for Medicare use your personal medical information to pay or deny your claims, to collect your premiums, to share your benefit payment with your other insurer(s), or to prepare your Medicare Summary Notice.
- Medicare may use your personal medical information to make sure you and other people with Medicare get quality health care, to provide customer service to you, to resolve any complaints you have, or to contact you about research studies.

Medicare may use or give out your personal medical information for the following purposes under limited circumstances:

- To state and other Federal agencies that have the legal right to receive Medicare data (such as to make sure Medicare is making proper payments and to assist Federal/state Medicaid programs)
- For public health activities (such as reporting disease outbreaks)
- For government health care oversight activities (such as fraud and abuse investigations)
- For judicial and administrative proceedings (such as in response to a court order)
- For law enforcement purposes (such as providing limited information to locate a missing person)
- For research studies, including surveys, that meet all privacy law requirements (such as research related to the prevention of disease or disability)
- To avoid a serious and imminent threat to health or safety
- To contact you about new or changed coverage under Medicare
- To create a collection of information that can no longer be traced back to you

By law, Medicare must have your written permission (an "authorization") to use or give out your personal medical information for any purpose that isn't set out in this notice. You may take back ("revoke") your written permission anytime, except to the extent that Medicare has already acted based on your permission.

By law, you have the right to take these actions:

- See and get a copy of your personal medical information held by Medicare.

- Have your personal medical information amended if you believe that it is wrong or if information is missing, and Medicare agrees. If Medicare disagrees, you may have a statement of your disagreement added to your personal medical information.

- Get a listing of those getting your personal medical information from Medicare. The listing won't cover your personal medical information that was given to you or your personal representative, that was given out to pay for your health care or for Medicare operations, or that was given out for law enforcement purposes if it would likely get in the way of these purposes.

- Ask Medicare to communicate with you in a different manner or at a different place (for example, by sending materials to a P.O. Box instead of your home address).

- Ask Medicare to limit how your personal medical information is used and given out to pay your claims and run the Medicare Program. Please note that Medicare may not be able to agree to your request.

- Get a separate paper copy of this notice.

Visit www.medicare.gov for more information on the following:

- Exercising your rights set out in this notice.

- Filing a complaint, if you believe Original Medicare has violated these privacy rights. Filing a complaint won't affect your coverage under Medicare.

You can also call 1-800-MEDICARE (1-800-633-4227) to get this information. Ask to speak to a customer service representative about Medicare's privacy notice. TTY users should call 1-877-486-2048.

You may file a complaint with the Secretary of the Department of Health and Human Services. Call the Office for Civil Rights at 1-800-368-1019. TTY users should call 1-800-537-7697. You can also visit www.hhs.gov/ocr/privacy.

By law, Medicare is required to follow the terms in this privacy notice. Medicare has the right to change the way your personal medical information is used and given out. If Medicare makes any changes to the way your personal medical information is used and given out, you will get a new notice by mail within 60 days of the change.

The Notice of Privacy Practices for Original Medicare became effective April 14, 2003.

Note: If you join a Medicare plan, the plan will let you know how it will use and release your personal information as permitted or required by law including for treatment, payment, health care operations, and for research and other purposes.

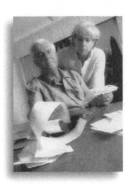

Protect Yourself from Identity Theft

Identity theft is a serious crime. Identity theft happens when someone uses your personal information without your consent to commit fraud or other crimes. Personal information includes things like your name and your Social Security, Medicare, or credit card numbers. Guard against identity theft by keeping your personal information safe.

If you think someone is using your personal information without your consent, call your local police department and the Federal Trade Commission's ID Theft Hotline at 1-877-438-4338 to make a report. TTY users should call 1-866-653-4261.

What You Can Do

Generally, no one should call you or come to your home uninvited to get you to join a Medicare plan. Don't give your personal information to someone who does this. **Only give personal information like your Medicare number to doctors, other health care providers, and plans approved by Medicare; any insurer who pays benefits on your behalf; and to trusted people in the community who work with Medicare, like your State Health Insurance Assistance Program (SHIP) or Social Security.** Call 1-800-MEDICARE (1-800-633-4227) if you aren't sure if a provider is approved by Medicare. TTY users should call 1-877-486-2048.

Plans Must Follow Rules

Medicare plans must follow certain rules when marketing their plans and getting your enrollment information. They can't ask you for credit card or banking information over the phone or via email, unless you're already a member of that plan. Medicare plans can't enroll you into a plan over the phone unless you call them and ask to enroll. **Call 1-800-MEDICARE to report any plans that ask for your personal information over the phone or that call to enroll you in a plan.** You can also call the Medicare Drug Integrity Contractor (MEDIC) at 1-877-7SAFERX (1-877-772-3379). The MEDIC helps prevent inappropriate activity and fights fraud, waste, and abuse in Medicare Advantage Plans (Part C) and Medicare Prescription Drug (Part D) Programs. For more information on the rules that Medicare plans must follow, visit www.medicare.gov/publications to view the booklet "Protecting Medicare and You from Fraud." You can also call 1-800-MEDICARE to find out if a copy can be mailed to you.

For more information about identity theft or to file a complaint online, visit www.ftc.gov/idtheft. You can also visit www.stopmedicarefraud.gov.

The Senior Medicare Patrol (SMP) Program Can Help You

The SMP Program educates and empowers people with Medicare to take an active role in detecting and preventing health care fraud and abuse. The SMP Program not only protects people with Medicare, it also helps preserve Medicare. There is an SMP Program in every state, the District of Columbia, Guam, the U.S. Virgin Islands, and Puerto Rico. Contact your local SMP Program to get personalized counseling and to find out about community events in your area. For more information or to find your local SMP Program, visit www.smpresource.org or call 1-877-808-2468. You can also call 1-800-MEDICARE (1-800-633-4227). TTY users should call 1-877-486-2048.

Protect Yourself and Medicare from Fraud

Blue words in the text are defined on pages 141–144.

Most doctors, pharmacists, plans, and other health care providers who work with Medicare are honest. Unfortunately, there may be some who are dishonest. Medicare fraud happens when Medicare is billed for services or supplies you never got. Medicare fraud costs Medicare a lot of money each year. You pay for it with higher premiums.

Remember these tips to help prevent billing fraud:

- Ask questions! You have the right to know everything about your health care, including the costs of the items and services billed to Medicare.
- Educate yourself about Medicare. Know your rights and what a provider can and can't bill to Medicare.
- Review your Medicare Summary Notice and other statements, and, if necessary, ask your health care provider about what items and services they have billed.
- Be wary of providers who tell you that the item or service isn't usually covered, but they "know how to bill Medicare" so Medicare will pay.

If you believe a Medicare plan or provider has used false information to mislead you, call 1-800-MEDICARE.

Protect Yourself and Medicare from Fraud (continued)

When you get health care services, record the dates on a calendar and save the receipts and statements you get from providers to check for mistakes. These include the Medicare Summary Notice (MSN) if you have Original Medicare, or similar statements that list the services you got or prescriptions you filled.

If you think you see an error or are billed for services you didn't get, do the following to find out what was billed:

- Ask your health care provider or supplier for an itemized statement. They should give this to you within 30 days.

- Check your MSN if you have Original Medicare to see if the service was billed to Medicare. If you're in a Medicare plan, check with your plan.

- Visit www.MyMedicare.gov to view your Medicare claims if you have Original Medicare. Your claims are generally available online within 24 hours after processing. The sooner you see and report errors, the sooner we can stop fraud. You can also call 1-800-MEDICARE (1-800-633-4227). TTY users should call 1-877-486-2048.

If you suspect there is a billing error, contact your health care provider to be sure the bill is correct. If you suspect fraud, call 1-800-MEDICARE.

For more information on protecting yourself from Medicare fraud and tips for spotting and reporting fraud, visit www.stopmedicarefraud.gov or contact your local SMP Program. See page 117.

Blue words in the text are defined on pages 141–144.

Fighting Fraud Can Pay

You may get a reward of up to $1,000 if you meet **all** these conditions:

- You report suspected Medicare fraud (for example, by calling 1-800-MEDICARE).

- The suspected Medicare fraud you report must be proven as potential fraud by the Program Safeguard Contractor, the Zone Program Integrity Contractor, or the Medicare Drug Integrity Contractor (the Medicare contractors that investigate potential fraud and abuse) and formally referred as part of a case by one of the contractors to the Office of Inspector General for further investigation.

- You aren't an "excluded individual." For example, you didn't participate in the fraud offense being reported. Or, there isn't another reward that you qualify for under another government program.

- The person or organization you're reporting isn't already under investigation by law enforcement.

- Your report leads to the recovery of at least $100 of Medicare money.

For more information, call 1-800-MEDICARE (1-800-633-4227). TTY users should call 1-877-486-2048.

Investigating Fraud Takes Time

We take all reports of suspected fraud seriously. When you report fraud, you may not hear of an outcome right away. It takes time to investigate your report and build a case.

How Medicare Protects You

With help from honest health care providers, suppliers, law enforcement, other government agencies, and citizens like you, Medicare is improving its ability to prevent fraud and protect you from identity theft.

The Department of Justice and the Department of Health and Human Services' Medicare Fraud Strike Force is a multi-agency team of Federal, state, and local investigators designed to combat Medicare fraud through Medicare data analysis and community policing. These agencies are also working together to both prevent fraud and enforce current anti-fraud laws around the country on a Health Care Fraud Prevention and Enforcement Action Team (HEAT). Over a 5-year period, it's estimated that the anti-fraud efforts and oversight will save $2.7 billion.

Because of all of these efforts, some dishonest health care providers have been removed from Medicare and some have gone to jail. These actions are saving money for taxpayers and protecting Medicare for the future.

Blue words in the text are defined on pages 141–144.

Reporting Suspected Medicaid Fraud

You can report Medicaid fraud to your State Medical Assistance (Medicaid) office. Visit www.cms.gov/fraudabuseforconsumers to learn more. Medicaid fraud can also be reported to the OIG National Fraud hotline at 1-800-HHS-TIPS (1-800-447-8477).

You're Protected from Discrimination

Every company or agency that works with Medicare must obey the law. You can't be treated differently because of your race, color, national origin, disability, age, religion, or sex. If you think that you haven't been treated fairly for any of these reasons, call the Department of Health and Human Services, Office for Civil Rights toll-free at 1-800-368-1019. TTY users should call 1-800-537-7697. You can also visit www.hhs.gov/ocr for more information.

The Medicare Beneficiary Ombudsman

An "ombudsman" is a person who reviews complaints and helps resolve them. The Medicare Beneficiary Ombudsman makes sure information about the following is available to all people with Medicare:

- Your Medicare coverage
- Information to help you make good health care decisions
- Your Medicare rights and protections
- How you can get issues resolved

The Ombudsman reviews the concerns raised by people with Medicare through 1-800-MEDICARE and through your State Health Insurance Assistance Program (SHIP).

Visit www.medicare.gov/ombudsman/resources.asp for information on inquiries and complaints, activities of the Ombudsman, and what people with Medicare need to know.

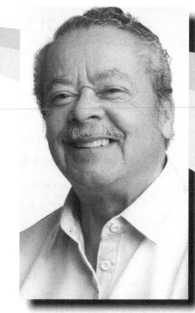

Planning Ahead

Section 6 includes information about the following:

Plan for Long-Term Care

Long-term care includes medical and non-medical care for people who have a chronic illness or disability. Non-medical care includes non-skilled personal care assistance, such as help with everyday activities, like dressing, bathing, and using the bathroom. At least 70% of people over 65 will need long-term care services at some point. **Medicare and most health insurance plans, including Medicare Supplement Insurance (Medigap) policies don't pay for this type of care, also called "custodial care."** Medicare only pays for medically-necessary skilled nursing facility care or home health care if you meet certain conditions. Long-term care can be provided at home, in the community, in assisted living, or in a nursing home. It's important to start planning for long-term care now to maintain your independence and to make sure you get the care you may need in the future.

Blue words in the text are defined on pages 141–144.

Paying for Long-Term Care

Long-term Care Insurance—This type of private insurance policy can help pay for many types of long-term care, including both skilled and non-skilled (custodial) care. Long-term care insurance can vary widely. Some policies may cover only nursing home care. Others may include coverage for a range of services, like adult day care, assisted living, medical equipment, and informal home care.

Note: Long-term care insurance doesn't replace your Medicare coverage.

Your current or former employer or union may offer long-term care insurance. Current and retired Federal employees, active and retired members of the uniformed services, and their qualified relatives can apply for coverage under the Federal Long-term Care Insurance Program. If you have questions, visit www.opm.gov/insure/ltc, or call the Federal Long-term Care Insurance Program at 1-800-582-3337. TTY users should call 1-800-843-3557.

Personal Resources—You can use your savings to pay for long-term care. Some insurance companies let you use your life insurance policy to pay for long-term care. Ask your insurance agent how this works.

Other Private Options—Besides long-term care insurance and personal resources, you may choose to pay for long-term care through a trust or annuity. The best option for you depends on your age, health status, risk of needing long-term care, and your personal financial situation. Visit www.longtermcare.gov for more information about your options.

Paying for Long-Term Care (continued)

Medicaid—Medicaid is a joint Federal and state program that pays for certain health services for people with limited income and resources. If you qualify, you may be able to get help to pay for nursing home care or other health care costs. See page 103 for more information about Medicaid.

Home and Community-based Services Programs—If you're already eligible for Medicaid (or, in some states, would be eligible for Medicaid coverage in a nursing home), you or your family members may be able to get help with the costs of services that help you stay in your home instead of moving to a nursing home. Examples include homemaker services, personal care, and respite care. For more information, contact your State Medical Assistance (Medicaid) office. Visit www.medicare.gov/contacts or call 1-800-MEDICARE (1-800-633-4227), and say "Medicaid" to get the phone number. TTY users should call 1-877-486-2048.

Veterans' Benefits—The Department of Veterans Affairs (VA) may provide long-term care for service-related disabilities or for certain eligible veterans. The VA also has a Housebound and an Aid and Attendance Allowance Program that provides cash grants to eligible disabled veterans and surviving spouses instead of formally-provided homemaker, personal care, and other services needed for help at home. For more information, call the VA at 1-800-827-1000, or visit www.va.gov.

Programs of All-inclusive Care for the Elderly (PACE)—PACE is a Medicare and Medicaid program offered in many states that allows people who otherwise need a nursing home-level of care to remain in the community. See page 83 for more information.

New—The Community Living Assistance Services and Supports (CLASS) Program will be a national, voluntary insurance program to help pay for services and supports needed to live as independently as possible. CLASS isn't available yet. Eligible working adults will be able to enroll in the CLASS program when it begins. Enrollees who meet certain eligibility requirements (including at least a 5-year vesting period and the need for assistance with activities of daily living) will have access to the benefit. Visit www.healthcare.gov to learn more.

Paying for Long-Term Care (continued)

Long-Term Care Contacts

Use the following resources to get more information about long-term care:

Blue words in the text are defined on pages 141–144.

- Visit www.medicare.gov/ltcplanning. You can visit www.medicare.gov/nhcompare to compare nursing homes or www.medicare.gov/hhcompare to compare home health agencies in your area.

- Call 1-800-MEDICARE (1-800-633-4227). TTY users should call 1-877-486-2048.

- Visit www.longtermcare.gov to learn more about planning for long-term care.

- Call your State Insurance Department to get information about long-term care insurance. Call 1-800-MEDICARE to get the phone number. You can also call your State Health Insurance Assistance Program. See pages 137–140 for their phone number.

- Call the National Association of Insurance Commissioners at 1-866-470-6242 to get a copy of "A Shopper's Guide to Long-term Care Insurance."

- Visit the Eldercare Locator, a public service of the U.S. Administration on Aging, at www.eldercare.gov to find your local Aging and Disability Resource Center (ADRC). You can also call 1-800-677-1116. ADRCs offer a full range of long-term care services and support in a single, coordinated program.

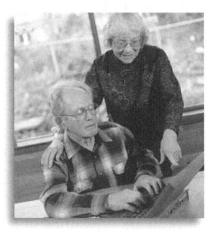

Advance Directives

Advance directives are legal documents that allow you to put in writing what kind of health care you would want or name someone who can speak for you if you were too ill to speak for yourself. Advance directives most often include the following:

- A health care proxy (durable power of attorney)
- A living will
- After-death wishes

Talking with your family, friends, and health care providers about your wishes is important, but these legal documents help ensure your wishes are followed. It's better to think about these important decisions before you're ill or a crisis strikes.

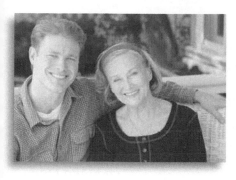

A health care proxy (sometimes called a "durable power of attorney for health care") is used to name the person you want to make health care decisions for you if you aren't able to make them yourself. Having a health care proxy is important because if you suddenly aren't able to make your own health care decisions, someone you trust will be able to make these decisions for you.

A living will is another way to make sure your voice is heard. It states which medical treatment you would accept or refuse if your life is threatened. Dialysis for kidney failure, a breathing machine if you can't breathe on your own, CPR (cardiopulmonary resuscitation) if your heart and breathing stop, or tube feeding if you can no longer eat are examples of such medical treatments.

In some states, advance directives can also include after-death wishes. These may include choices such as organ and tissue donation.

Advance Directives (continued)

If you already have advance directives, take time now to review them to be sure you're still satisfied with your decisions and your health care proxy is still willing and able to carry out your plans. Find out how to cancel or update them in your state if they no longer reflect your wishes. Each state has its own laws for creating advance directives. Some states may allow you to combine your advance directives in one document. For more information, contact your health care provider, an attorney, your local Area Agency on Aging, or your state health department.

Tips If You Choose to Have Advanced Directives

1. Keep the original copies of your advance directives where they are easily found.

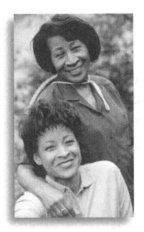

2. Give the person you've named as your health care proxy, and others close to you, a copy of your advance directives.

3. Give your doctor or other health care provider a copy of your advance directives for your medical record. Provide a copy to a hospital or nursing home you stay in or any ambulatory surgical center where you have procedures done.

4. Carry a card in your wallet that states you have advance directives.

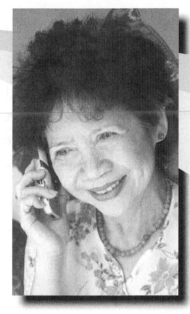

Helpful Resources and Tools

Section 7 includes information about the following:

If you have a question or complaint about the quality of a Medicare-covered service, call your local Quality Improvement Organization (QIO). Visit www.medicare.gov/contacts to get your QIO's phone number. You can also call 1-800-MEDICARE (1-800-633-4227). TTY users should call 1-877-486-2048.

1-800-MEDICARE (1-800-633-4227)
TTY Users Call 1-877-486-2048

Get Information 24 Hours a Day, Including Weekends.

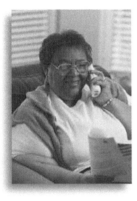

- Speak clearly, have your Medicare card in front of you, and be ready to provide your Medicare number. This helps reduce the amount of time you may wait to speak to a customer service representative. It also allows us to play messages that may specifically impact your coverage and may help us get you to a representative more quickly.

- To enter your Medicare number, speak the numbers and letters clearly one at a time. Or, enter your Medicare number on the phone keypad. Use the star key to indicate any place there may be a letter. For example, if your Medicare number is 000-00-0000A, you would enter 0-0-0-0-0-0-0-0-0-*. The voice system will then ask you for that letter.

- **Say "Agent" at anytime to talk to a customer service representative, or use this chart**. If you need help in a language other than English or Spanish, let the customer service representative know the language so you can get free translation services.

If you're calling about...	Say ...
Medicare prescription drug coverage	"Drug Coverage"
Claim or billing issues, or appeals	"Claims" or "Billing"
Preventive services	"Preventive Services"
Help paying health or prescription drug costs	"Limited Income"
Forms or publications	"Publications"
Phone numbers for your State Medical Assistance (Medicaid) office	"Medicaid"
Outpatient doctor's care	"Doctor Service"
Hospital visit or emergency room care	"Hospital Stay"
Equipment or supplies like oxygen, wheelchairs, walkers, or diabetic supplies	"Medical Supplies"
Information about your Part B deductible	"Deductible"
Nursing home services	"Nursing Home"

1-800-MEDICARE (1-800-633-4227) (continued)

People who get benefits from the Railroad Retirement Board should call 1-800-833-4455 with questions about Part B services and bills.

> If you want someone to be able to call 1-800-MEDICARE on your behalf, you need to let Medicare know in writing. You can fill out a "Medicare Authorization to Disclose Personal Health Information" form so Medicare can give your personal health information to someone other than you. You can do this by visiting www.medicare.gov/medicareonlineforms or by calling 1-800-MEDICARE (1-800-633-4227) to get a copy of the form. TTY users should call 1-877-486-2048. You may want to do this now in case you become unable to do it later.

State Health Insurance Assistance Programs (SHIPs)

SHIPs are state programs that get money from the Federal government to give free local health insurance counseling to people with Medicare. SHIPs are independent and not connected to any insurance company or health plan. SHIP volunteers work hard to help you with the following Medicare questions or concerns:
- Your Medicare rights
- Complaints about your medical care or treatment
- Billing problems
- Plan choices

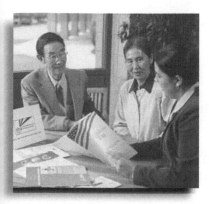

See pages 137–140 for the phone number of your local SHIP. If you would like to become a volunteer SHIP counselor, contact the SHIP in your state to learn more.

Go Online to Get the Information You Need

Need General Information about Medicare?

Visit www.medicare.gov:

- Get detailed information about the Medicare health and prescription drug plans in your area, including what they cost and what services they provide.
- Find doctors or other health care providers and suppliers who participate in Medicare.
- See what Medicare covers, including preventive services.
- Get Medicare appeals information and forms.
- Get information about the quality of care provided by plans, nursing homes, hospitals, home health agencies, and dialysis facilities.
- Look up helpful Web sites and phone numbers.

Need Personalized Medicare Information?

Register at www.MyMedicare.gov, Medicare's secure online service for accessing your personal Medicare information:

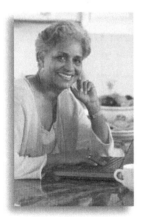

- Create and print an "On the Go" report that lists information you can share with your providers.
- Add or change information such as health conditions and allergies.
- View or change your personal drug list and pharmacy information, and see your prescription drug costs.
- Search for and create a list of your favorite providers, and access quality information about them.
- Complete your Initial Enrollment Questionnaire so your bills can get paid correctly.
- Track Original Medicare claims, and order a Medicare Summary Notice.
- Check your Part B deductible status.

Need Help Finding Other Health Insurance Options?

Visit www.healthcare.gov:

- Take control of your health care with new information and resources that will help you access quality and affordable health coverage.
- Find public and private health coverage options tailored for your needs in a single easy to use tool.

Compare the Quality of Plans and Providers

You can't always plan ahead when you need health care, but when you can, take time to compare. Medicare collects information about the quality and safety of medical care and services given by most Medicare plans and other health care providers. Medicare also has information about the experiences of people with the care and services they get.

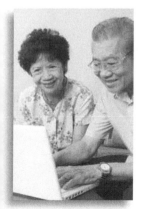

Blue words in the text are defined on pages 141–144.

Compare the quality of care (how well plans and providers work to give you the best care possible) and services given by health and prescription drug plans or health care providers nationwide by visiting www.medicare.gov or by calling your State Health Insurance Assistance Program (SHIP). See pages 137–140 for the phone number.

When you, a family member, friend, or SHIP counselor visit Medicare's Web site, under "Resource Locator," select one of the following:

- "Drug and Health Plans"
- "Dialysis Facilities"
- "Home Health Agencies"
- "Hospitals"
- "Nursing Homes"

These search tools on www.medicare.gov give you a "snapshot" of the quality of care and services some plans and providers give. Find out more about the quality of care and services by doing the following:

- Ask what your plan or provider does to ensure and improve the quality of care and services. Every plan and health care provider should have someone you can talk to about quality.
- Ask your doctor or other health care provider what he or she thinks about the quality of care or services the plan or other providers give. You can also talk to your doctor or other health care provider about Medicare's information on quality of care and services.

Medicare is Working to Better Coordinate Your Care

Medicare continues to look for ways to better coordinate your care and to make sure that you get the best health care possible. Health information technology (also called Health IT) and improved ways to deliver your care can help manage your health information, improve how you communicate with your health care providers, and improve the quality and coordination of your health care. These tools also reduce paperwork, medical errors, and health care costs.

Here are examples of how your **health care providers** can better coordinate your care:

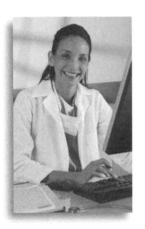

Electronic Health Records (EHRs)—A safe and confidential record that your doctor, other health care provider, medical office staff, or a hospital keeps on a computer about your health care or treatments. If your providers use electronic health records, they can join a network to securely share your records with each other.

- EHRs can help lower the chances of medical errors, eliminate duplicate tests, and may improve your overall quality of care.
- EHRs can help your providers have the same up-to-date information about your conditions, treatments, tests, and prescriptions.

Medicare is Working to Better Coordinate Your Care (continued)

Electronic Prescribing—An electronic way for your prescribers (your doctor or other health care provider who is legally allowed to write prescriptions) to send your prescriptions directly to your pharmacy. Electronic prescribing can save you money, time, and help keep you safe.

- You don't have to drop off and wait for your pharmacist to fill your prescription. Your prescription may be ready when you arrive.
- Prescribers can check which drugs your insurance covers and prescribe a drug that costs you less.
- Electronic prescriptions are easier for the pharmacist to read than handwritten prescriptions. This means there's less chance that you will get the wrong drug or dose.
- Prescribers will have secure access to your prescription history, so they can be alerted to potential drug interactions, allergies, and other warnings.

EHRs can also help you get the following important information quickly:

- Details describing your health conditions and treatments you discussed with your provider.
- An explanation of medical terms and test results found in your record.

NEW: Accountable Care Organizations (ACOs)—Starting in 2012, if you have Original Medicare, your doctor may choose to join an Accountable Care Organization (ACO). This is a team of health care providers that agree to work together to improve the overall

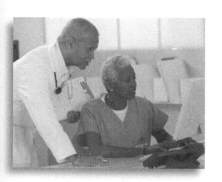

quality, cost, and care of patients. An ACO **won't** affect your costs, benefits, or coverage. You can still choose your doctor. If your doctor belongs to an ACO, you can continue getting care from your doctor. Or, you can choose to see a doctor who doesn't participate in the ACO. For more information, visit www.medicare.gov or call 1-800-MEDICARE (1-800-633-4227). TTY users should call 1-877-486-2048.

You Can Manage Your Health Information Online

Here's what **you** can do to help manage your health information:

Personal Health Records (PHRs)—A record with information about your health that you or someone helping you keeps for easy reference using a computer.

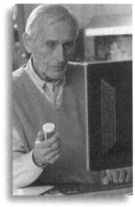

- These easy to use tools can help you manage your health information from anywhere you have Internet access.
- With a PHR, you can keep track of health information, like the date of your last physical, major illnesses, operations, allergies, or a list of your prescriptions.
- PHRs are often offered by providers, health plans, and private companies. Some are free, while others charge fees.
- When you use a PHR, make sure that it's on a secure Web site. With a secure Web site, you usually have to create a unique user ID and password, and the information you type is encrypted (put in code) so other people can't read it.

There are Federal and state laws that protect the privacy and security of your information. PHRs that aren't sponsored or maintained by health plans or health care providers may not have privacy rules.

Visit www.medicare.gov/phr to learn more about Personal Health Records.

You Can Manage Your Health Information Online (continued)

NEW: Medicare's "Blue Button"—MyMedicare.gov has a new "Blue Button" feature that lets you download your Original Medicare claims. The Blue Button also allows you to enter information such as emergency contacts, names of pharmacies and providers, self-reported allergies, medical conditions, and prescription drugs.

After logging on to the secure www.MyMedicare.gov site, you can click the Blue Button and download a computer file of your claims data and add personal health information that you can share with health care providers, caregivers, and family members.

- Having access to information from Medicare claims and self-entered personal health information can help you better understand your medical history and partner more effectively with providers.

- The Blue Button data file can also be imported into other health management tools, such as one of the PHR tools described on page 134. To find a PHR that can upload the blue button file, visit www.myphr.com.

- The Blue Button is safe, secure, reliable, and easy to use.

Visit www.MyMedicare.gov to sign up for your account and use the Blue Button today!

Medicare Publications

To read, print, or download copies of booklets, brochures, or fact sheets on different Medicare topics, visit www.medicare.gov/publications. You can search by keyword (such as "rights" or "mental health"), or select "View All Publications."

If the publication you want has a check box after "Order Publication," you can have a printed copy mailed to you. You can also call 1-800-MEDICARE (1-800-633-4227) and say "Publications" to find out if a printed copy can be mailed to you. TTY users should call 1-877-486-2048.

Some publications are also available as podcasts that you can download and listen to.

Blue words in the text are defined on pages 141–144.

Caregiver Resources

Do You Help Someone With Medicare?

Medicare has resources to help you get the information you need.

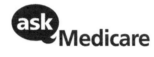

- Visit "Ask Medicare" at www.medicare.gov/caregivers to help someone you care for choose a drug plan, compare nursing homes, get help with billing, and more.

- Sign up for the free bi-monthly "Ask Medicare" electronic newsletter (e-Newsletter) when you go to www.medicare.gov/caregivers. The e-Newsletter has the latest information including important dates, Medicare changes, and resources in your community.

- Visit the Eldercare Locator, a public service of the U.S. Administration on Aging, at www.eldercare.gov, or call 1-800-677-1116 to find caregiver support services in your area.

- The Centers for Medicare & Medicaid Services (CMS) is now on Twitter! Follow official Medicare information at @CMSGov and the Children's Health Insurance Program at @IKNGov.

- Visit www.YouTube.com/cmshhsgov to see videos covering different health care topics on Medicare's YouTube channel.

State Health Insurance Assistance Programs (SHIPs)

For help with questions about appeals, buying other insurance, choosing a health plan, buying a Medigap policy, and Medicare rights and protections.

This page has been intentionally left blank. The printed version contains phone number information. For the most recent phone number information, please visit www.medicare.gov/contacts/home.asp. Thank you.

This page has been intentionally left blank. The printed version contains phone number information. For the most recent phone number information, please visit www.medicare.gov/contacts/home.asp. Thank you.

This page has been intentionally left blank. The printed version contains phone number information. For the most recent phone number information, please visit www.medicare.gov/contacts/home.asp. Thank you.

This page has been intentionally left blank. The printed version contains phone number information. For the most recent phone number information, please visit www.medicare.gov/contacts/home.asp. Thank you.

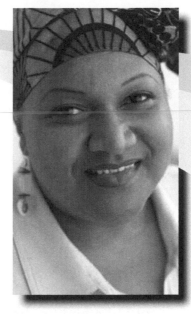

Definitions

Assignment—An agreement by your doctor, other health care provider, or supplier to be paid directly by Medicare, to accept the payment amount Medicare approves for the service, and not to bill you for any more than the Medicare deductible and coinsurance.

Benefit Period—The way that Original Medicare measures your use of hospital and skilled nursing facility (SNF) services. A benefit period begins the day you are admitted as an inpatient in a hospital or skilled nursing facility. The benefit period ends when you haven't received any inpatient hospital care (or skilled care in a SNF) for 60 days in a row. If you go into a hospital or a skilled nursing facility after one benefit period has ended, a new benefit period begins. You must pay the inpatient hospital deductible for each benefit period. There is no limit to the number of benefit periods.

Coinsurance—An amount you may be required to pay as your share of the cost for services after you pay any deductibles. Coinsurance is usually a percentage (for example, 20%).

Copayment—An amount you may be required to pay as your share of the cost for a medical service or supply, like a doctor's visit, hospital outpatient visit, or prescription. A copayment is usually a set amount, rather than a percentage. For example, you might pay $10 or $20 for a doctor's visit or prescription.

Creditable Prescription Drug Coverage—Prescription drug coverage (for example, from an employer or union) that's expected to pay, on average, at least as much as Medicare's standard prescription drug coverage. People who have this kind of coverage when they become eligible for Medicare can generally keep that coverage without paying a penalty, if they decide to enroll in Medicare prescription drug coverage later.

Critical Access Hospital—A small facility that provides outpatient services, as well as inpatient services on a limited basis, to people in rural areas.

Custodial Care—Nonskilled personal care, such as help with activities of daily living like bathing, dressing, eating, getting in or out of a bed or chair, moving around, and using the bathroom. It may also include the kind of health-related care that most people do themselves, like using eye drops. In most cases, Medicare doesn't pay for custodial care.

Deductible—The amount you must pay for health care or prescriptions before Original Medicare, your prescription drug plan, or your other insurance begins to pay.

Extra Help—A Medicare program to help people with limited income and resources pay Medicare prescription drug program costs, such as premiums, deductibles, and coinsurance.

Formulary—A list of prescription drugs covered by a prescription drug plan or another insurance plan offering prescription drug benefits.

Inpatient Rehabilitation Facility—A hospital, or part of a hospital, that provides an intensive rehabilitation program to inpatients.

Institution—For the purposes of this publication, an institution is a facility that provides short term or long term care, such as a nursing home, skilled nursing facility (SNF), or rehabilitation hospital. Private residences, such as an assisted living facility or group home, aren't considered institutions for this purpose.

Lifetime Reserve Days—In Original Medicare, these are additional days that Medicare will pay for when you're in a hospital for more than 90 days. You have a total of 60 reserve days that can be used during your lifetime. For each lifetime reserve day, Medicare pays all covered costs except for a daily coinsurance.

Long-Term Care—A variety of services that help people with their medical and non-medical needs over a period of time. Long-term care can be provided at home, in the community, or in various other types of facilities, including nursing homes and assisted living facilities. Most long-term care is custodial care. Medicare doesn't pay for this type of care if this is the only kind of care you need.

Long-Term Care Hospital—Acute care hospitals that provide treatment for patients who stay, on average, more than 25 days. Most patients are transferred from an intensive or critical care unit. Services provided include comprehensive rehabilitation, respiratory therapy, head trauma treatment, and pain management.

Medically Necessary—Services or supplies that are needed for the diagnosis or treatment of your medical condition and meet accepted standards of medical practice.

Medicare-Approved Amount—In Original Medicare, this is the amount a doctor or supplier that accepts assignment can be paid. It may be less than the actual amount a doctor or supplier charges. Medicare pays part of this amount and you're responsible for the difference.

Medicare Health Plan—A plan offered by a private company that contracts with Medicare to provide Part A and Part B benefits to people with Medicare who enroll in the plan. Medicare Health Plans include all Medicare Advantage Plans, Medicare Cost Plans, Demonstration/Pilot Programs, and Programs of All-inclusive Care for the Elderly (PACE).

Medicare Plan—Refers to any way other than Original Medicare that you can get your Medicare health or prescription drug coverage. This term includes all Medicare health plans and Medicare Prescription Drug Plans.

Premium—The periodic payment to Medicare, an insurance company, or a health care plan for health or prescription drug coverage.

Preventive Services—Health care to prevent illness or detect illness at an early stage, when treatment is likely to work best (for example, preventive services include Pap tests, flu shots, and screening mammograms).

Primary Care Doctor—Your primary care doctor is the doctor you see first for most health problems. He or she makes sure you get the care you need to keep you healthy. He or she also may talk with other doctors and health care providers about your care and refer you to them. In many Medicare Advantage Plans, you must see your primary care doctor before you see any other health care provider.

Quality Improvement Organization (QIO)—A group of practicing doctors and other health care experts paid by the Federal government to check and improve the care given to people with Medicare.

Referral—A written order from your primary care doctor for you to see a specialist or to get certain medical services. In many Health Maintenance Organizations (HMOs), you need to get a referral before you can get medical care from anyone except your primary care doctor. If you don't get a referral first, the plan may not pay for the services.

Service Area—A geographic area where a health insurance plan accepts members if it limits membership based on where people live. For plans that limit which doctors and hospitals you may use, it's also generally the area where you can get routine (non-emergency) services. The plan may disenroll you if you move out of the plan's service area.

Skilled Nursing Facility (SNF) Care—Skilled nursing care and rehabilitation services provided on a continuous, daily basis, in a skilled nursing facility. Examples of skilled nursing facility care include physical therapy or intravenous injections that can only be given by a registered nurse or doctor.

TTY—A teletypewriter (TTY) is a communication device used by people who are deaf, hard-of-hearing, or have a severe speech impairment. People who don't have a TTY can communicate with a TTY user through a message relay center (MRC). An MRC has TTY operators available to send and interpret TTY messages.

Notes

Want to Save?

Extra Help is available!

Many people qualify to get Extra Help paying their Medicare prescription drug costs but don't know it. Most people who qualify and join a Medicare drug plan will pay no more than $6.50 for brand-name drugs and $2.60 for generics. Don't miss out on a chance to save. Extra Help and other programs (like Medicare Savings Programs) may help make your health care and prescription drug costs more affordable. See pages 98–104 for more information about Extra Help and other programs.

Choose to get future handbooks electronically.

Save tax dollars and help the environment by signing up to get your future "Medicare & You" handbooks electronically (also called the "eHandbook"). Visit www.MyMedicare.gov to request eHandbooks. We'll send you an email next September when the new eHandbook is available. You won't get a printed copy of your handbook in the mail if you choose to get it electronically.

Did your household get more than one copy of "Medicare & You?"

This may happen if there is a slight difference in how your or your spouse's address is entered in Social Security's or the Railroad Retirement Board's (RRB) mailing system. If you want to get only one copy in the future, call 1-800-MEDICARE (1-800-633-4227), and say "Agent." TTY users should call 1-877-486-2048. If you get RRB benefits, call your local RRB office or 1-877-772-5772.

Part A and Part B Costs

The law requires Medicare to send the information in this handbook to all people with Medicare 15 days before the start of the fall Open Enrollment Period. The 2012 premium and deductible amounts for Part A and Part B weren't available to include at the time of printing. To get the most up-to-date information on these costs, visit www.medicare.gov or call 1-800-MEDICARE (1-800-633-4227). TTY users should call 1-877-486-2048.

Part C and Part D (Medicare Health and Prescription Drug Plans) Costs for Covered Services and Supplies

Cost information for the Medicare plans in your area is available at www.medicare.gov. You can also contact the plan, or call 1-800-MEDICARE. You can also call your State Health Insurance Assistance Program (SHIP). See pages 137–140 for the phone number. Medicare Advantage Plans (like an HMO or PPO) must cover all Part A and Part B-covered services and supplies. Check your plan's materials for actual amounts.

Medicare cares about what you think. If you have general comments about this handbook, email us at medicareandyou@cms.hhs.gov. We can't respond to every comment, but we will consider your feedback when writing future versions.

**U.S. DEPARTMENT OF
HEALTH AND HUMAN SERVICES**

Centers for Medicare & Medicaid Services
7500 Security Boulevard
Baltimore, Maryland 21244-1850

Official Business
Penalty for Private Use, $300

CMS Product No. 10050
August 2011

National Medicare Handbook

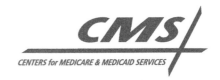

- Also available in Spanish, Braille, Audio CD, and Large Print (English and Spanish).
- New address? Call Social Security at 1-800-772-1213. TTY users should call 1-800-325-0778.

- ¿Necesita usted una copia de este manual en Español? Llame al 1-800-MEDICARE (1-800-633-4227). Los usuarios de TTY deberán llamar al 1-877-486-2048.

medicare
1-800-MEDICARE (1-800-633-4227)
TTY 1-877-486-2048

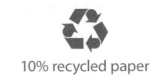

10% recycled paper

www.bnpublishing.com

CPSIA information can be obtained at www.ICGtesting.com
Printed in the USA
LVOW011552280113

317566LV00014B/558/P